CANCER, SEX, AND INTIMACY

Cancer, Sex, and Intimacy

A Couple's Guide

Anne Katz, PhD, RN

JOHNS HOPKINS UNIVERSITY PRESS

Baltimore

© 2026 Johns Hopkins University Press
All rights reserved. Published 2026
First printed in the United States of America on acid-free paper
9 8 7 6 5 4 3 2 1

Johns Hopkins University Press
2715 North Charles Street
Baltimore, Maryland 21218
www.press.jhu.edu

Library of Congress Cataloging-in-Publication Data is available.

ISBN 978-1-4214-5377-4 (hardcover)
ISBN 978-1-4214-5378-1 (paperback)
ISBN 978-1-4214-5379-8 (ebook)

A catalog record for this book is available from the British Library.

*Special discounts are available for bulk purchases of this book. For more
information, please contact Special Sales at specialsales@jh.edu.*

EU GPSR Authorized Representative
LOGOS EUROPE, 9 rue Nicolas Poussin,
17000, La Rochelle, France
E-mail: Contact@logoseurope.eu

For Alan
Forty-eight years and counting

Contents

Preface

This book and the stories within are based on my 20-plus years of clinical practice. While I've changed names and identifying characteristics to preserve the anonymity of the couples and their experiences described in each chapter, these descriptions are based on their real lives before, during, and after cancer.

In each story, you'll see sections that reflect evidence-based guidance as well as suggestions gleaned from my many years of experience as a registered nurse and certified sexuality counselor.

Writing this book has served as a reflective exercise for me, and I'm appreciative of the opportunity to remember couples I have cared for and about over the years. These memories have reminded me of the immense privilege granted to me by these couples who shared their experiences, both painful and joyful. I have learned so much from them about the loss of certainty that most of us have in what our lives will look like in the future, about the ability to cope with what was once unthinkable, and about the gift, for most, of unconditional support from a partner.

Most of all, I have seen the best of humanity, compassion, and love between two people, and for this I will also always be grateful.

CANCER, SEX, AND INTIMACY

Introduction

Human sexuality is a complex phenomenon. In part, it is based on the structure and function of sexual organs acting with and influenced by hormones. It also is connected to the brain through cognition, emotion, motivation, and memory. Sexuality—the way we see ourselves as sexual beings and whom we desire and love—is an important part of identity and quality of life across the lifespan.

Cancer and, more importantly, its treatment cause alterations in sexuality. The variety of treatments offered—surgery, radiation therapy, chemotherapy, and the new targeted immunotherapies—all have impacts on sexuality. Patients and their partners are often not informed of sexual side effects, and so when they happen, the response is shock, sadness, and often frustration in attempts to find information and help. It may also be that this information about side effects is provided at a time when patients and partners are unable to consider it (at the time of diagnosis of a life-threatening disease, for example), and the health-care provider does not talk about the topic again, thinking it has been discussed or is unnecessary or too uncomfortable to revisit.

People's views of themselves and others as sexual beings are influenced by cultural, ethnic, and religious beliefs and practices, as well as by knowledge of their own bodies and how they function. The definition of sexuality also encompasses people's relationships with others and how they are perceived by others as sexual beings. Sexuality is sometimes spoken of as intimacy, and the word "intimacy" in this case is used as a euphemism. Intimacy often is equated with privacy and closeness, but in the context of human interactions, intimacy involves self-disclosure, partner disclosure, and partner responsiveness—in essence, the connectedness between two people. This contrasts with sexual functioning, which is seen as what people do as sexual beings. Sexual dysfunction is said to exist when sexual activity or functioning does not follow some predetermined path and is seen as wrong, abnormal, or requiring intervention.

CANCER AND SEXUALITY

In the context of cancer, sexuality is an important aspect of quality of life, and cancer affects quality of life in multiple dimensions, including psychological, functional, social, and physical. The cancer itself may affect both sexuality and sexual functioning, and the many different treatment approaches have an impact on individuals, with physical, psychological, and social consequences. For many people newly diagnosed with cancer, the diagnosis may feel like a death sentence, and the meaning they ascribe to sexuality may be in stark contrast to this. For some, sexuality is something that is equated with health, life, and reproduction. To even think about sex when the threat of death looms seems antithetical; therefore, many give up on this aspect of their lives. Although the fight for survival is acute, sex itself, and even thinking of oneself as a sexual being, is relegated to the back burner. Sexual problems can result from psychological responses to the diagnosis and treatment. Cancer and its treatments can affect physical, endocrine, neurogenic, and vascular functioning. Consequences from any of the drugs used to treat the cancer or its side effects also may have an impact on sexual functioning.

STAGES OF ILLNESS

Any illness, including cancer, has different stages associated with it, and these stages affect sexuality and sexual functioning. Concerns about sexuality can occur at any stage of the cancer trajectory, from diagnosis to advanced and terminal cancer. They are often not considered to be "medical" concerns, however, and so they're not addressed. In the crisis phase, individuals with cancer must reorganize their lives and adapt to the crisis. Patients must learn to live with symptoms, adapt to treatments, and develop flexibility to the social demands of illness. In the chronic or survivorship phase of the illness, individuals must renegotiate relationships within the family, learn to live with uncertainty, and balance connectedness and separateness within social and familial relationships. The end-of-life phase requires individuals with cancer and their families to live with anticipatory grief.

It may take many months or years to recover from treatment and the physical and psychological changes that have occurred. Some survivors return to their previous level of sexual functioning; some do not. Coping with the sexual changes requires an adjustment about what constitutes sex and satisfaction. Changes made within the context of the couple's relationship, termed "flexible coping," are key to ongoing sexual engagement and satisfaction. Alterations in sexual functioning include decreases in sexual frequency, satisfaction, and participation in penetrative and nonpenetrative activities for women and men, and in all cancer types. Although physical factors such as erectile difficulties and vulvovaginal dryness are cited as significant reasons for these decreases, relationship factors are also important. These include relationship strain and abandonment, as well as the challenges of establishing new relationships after cancer. Psychological factors play a role too, including loss of masculine or feminine identity, sadness, frustration, feelings of inadequacy, and disappointment at the loss of sexual connection with a partner.

Many survivors do not know that help is available because they have never been asked whether they have experienced any changes, or they may not have revealed their concerns when asked. Whether this results in distress is extremely variable, and many survivors never seek help for dealing with sexual changes. But sexuality and sexual functioning are important to cancer survivors. Given the significant number of cancer survivors living among us, this is a substantial problem.

The aim of *Cancer, Sex, and Intimacy* is to educate and inform survivors and their partners at all stages of the disease about the sexual side effects and potential treatments through the use of stories of couples coping with these side effects. This introduction and the first chapter set the stage for understanding the anatomy (organs, blood vessels, and nerves) and physiology (how things work) of the sexual organs, including the brain—regarded as the largest sexual organ! Chapters 2 through 13 provide resources (books, websites, podcasts, etc.) to further the reader's ability to find help, if needed. Finally, two appendices are included that provide instructions for mindfulness meditation and sensate focus exercises.

The couples highlighted in these stories are compilations of patients and partners that I have provided education and counselling to over the course of more than two decades of clinical practice. I hope readers find their stories educational and encouraging.

CHAPTER 1

The Human Sexual Response

This chapter describes how men and women experience attraction, desire, and the wide range of sexual activity that humans explore and engage in. As preparation for the chapters that follow, I'll explain how cancer impacts this experience.

SEXUAL ANATOMY

The *external female sexual organs* are the vulva (clitoris, labia majora and minora) and the entrance to the vagina (called the "vaginal introitus"). Internally, the sex organs are the vagina and cervix, and the uterus and uterine tubes, as well as the ovaries. The ovaries are responsible for producing the hormones that influence sexual functioning and egg production. The breasts are secondary sex organs that grow and develop during puberty. Stimulation of the nipples and areolae for many women is important for sexual arousal.

All these structures are richly supplied with nerve endings and blood vessels, and respond to stimulation by swelling. The clitoris is equal to the male penis and is responsible for orgasms. The vagina extends internally upward and backward, and is approximately 3–5 inches in length. At rest, it is a collapsed tube whose walls touch one another along their length. The cervix is found at the top of the vagina and is the entry to the uterus.

The ovaries produce several hormones, including estrogen, progesterone, and testosterone, in varying amounts through the menstrual cycle. The ovaries, too, are where the eggs are stored and then released monthly prior to menopause, and they are necessary for conception.

The *external male sexual organs* are the penis and scrotum. The internal organs are the testicles, the vas deferens, the seminal vesicles, the Cowper glands, and the prostate. The scrotum is a sack of tissue containing the testicles and is covered with hair after puberty. The testicles are where sperm are stored and testosterone is produced. Sperm travel through two tubes (called the "vas deferens") into the prostate, where fluid is added; this is now called "semen" and is expelled to the outside of the body through the penis, a process called "ejaculation" that usually is accompanied by orgasm.

HORMONAL INFLUENCES

The hypothalamus and pituitary gland are found in the brain, and they regulate the secretion of hormones by the ovaries and testicles. The bodies of both men and women contain estrogen and testosterone but in different amounts, with men having more testosterone and less estrogen, and women having the opposite.

Estrogen is regarded as the hormone of arousal in women and is involved in the secretion of vaginal lubrication. After menopause, the ovarian production of estrogen diminishes significantly. Women produce a small amount of testosterone in the ovaries and in the adrenal glands (found over the kidneys). These hormones are involved in the growth of pubic hair and underarm hair. The relationship between hormones, especially testosterone, and desire is not confirmed by research, but testosterone together with estrogen is thought to be involved in what sensations are perceived by the brain to be sexual.

The primary male sex hormone is testosterone, which is produced in the testes and, to a lesser extent, by the adrenal glands over the kidneys. Testosterone is involved in the development of secondary sex characteristics (body hair and enlargement of the testicles and penis) as well as sperm production. Testosterone is responsible for sexual desire in men.

SEX AND THE BRAIN

Parts of the brain play key roles in sexual functioning. Cerebral cortex activation occurs when people experience sexual thoughts or fantasies. Signals sent to the sexual organs cause increased blood flow to the genitals (arousal). The cerebral cortex also interprets stimuli as sexually stimulating or not and judges whether sexual behavior is pleasurable.

THE SEXUAL RESPONSE CYCLE

Dr. William Masters and Virginia Johnson[1] were the first to describe the human sexual response. The *Masters and Johnson model* is a four-stage model with major similarities between men and women. The four stages of their model are excitement, plateau, orgasm, and resolution, representing episodes of blood flow to the genitals and breasts along with muscle contractions.

In the excitement (arousal) stage, heart rate and blood pressure increase, and blood flows into the tissues of the sexual organs. For *women*, the breasts enlarge in size, and a reddish flush may appear on the chest and neck. The nipples become more erect. Increased blood flow to the genital tissues results in swelling of the clitoris and vulvar structures. The upper two-thirds of the vagina grows bigger, and the walls secrete a fluid (vaginal lubrication). For men, the penis becomes erect as blood flow into the tissues and the scrotum moves upward into the body.

The plateau phase is a state of advanced arousal. Blood pressure and heart rate continue to increase, and breathing becomes rapid.

Orgasm is the phase of intense muscular contractions that are usually experienced as pleasurable for both men and women. In men this is usually accompanied by ejaculation of semen.

In the resolution phase, the body returns to its normal non-aroused state. For both men and women, muscle tension disappears and heart rate, blood pressure, and breathing return to normal. During this phase in women, blood moves out of the pelvic organs. In men, the penis loses its rigidity. For men, the resolution phase is followed by a period (called the "refractory period") during which ejaculation and orgasm are not possible. In young men, the refractory period may last a few minutes. But as men age, this period lasts longer, and older men may not be able to have another orgasm or ejaculation for hours or even days. Women do not experience a refractory period and may have multiple orgasms with continued stimulation.

Helen Singer Kaplan[2] introduced the idea of desire in her description of the human sexual response cycle. Her model comprises three parts: desire, excitement, and orgasm, closely modeled on the work of Masters and Johnson. According to Kaplan, the psychological processes of emotion and cognition that lead to the subjective feeling of desire are an important part of the sexual response cycle. Excitement in this model follows much the same process as in the Masters and Johnson model, with blood flow causing erections for men and arousal and lubrication for women. Orgasm is a series of muscular contractions; Kaplan does not talk about resolution in her model. Kaplan's model is not necessarily a linear process, such as the model suggested by Masters and Johnson. Kaplan describes her model as consisting of three independent phases; according to this model, it is possible to experience excitement without first experiencing desire.

Zilbergeld and Ellison[3] proposed a five-stage model that has both psychological and physiologic parts, which are mostly independent of one another. Their model contains the following phases:

- interest (similar to Kaplan)
- arousal (increased blood flow to the genitals, similar to Masters and Johnson)
- physiologic readiness (lubrication for women and erections for men)
- orgasm (muscle contractions and pleasurable sensations)
- satisfaction (psychological/cognitive reaction)

Rosemary Basson[4] focuses on the female sexual response cycle with a heavy emphasis on psychological and emotional processes, as opposed to the other models described. This model is circular rather than linear and describes responsive versus spontaneous desire. In her model, libido (desire) is said to occur at the same time as arousal. She suggests that women have many reasons to be receptive to or instigators of sexual activity. These include rewards such as emotional closeness, feelings of well-being, and lack of negative feelings resulting from avoiding sex. Sexual stimuli (for example her partner's touch) are processed psychologically and physically, and lead to feelings of arousal and a responsive feeling of desire, which usually occur at the same time. Sexual satisfaction for women is thought to further increase their motivation and willingness to be receptive in a future encounter. Satisfaction does not necessarily mean that the woman has an orgasm; for many women, the feelings of closeness or intimacy and knowing that one's partner may have achieved orgasm or satisfaction may be enough for her satisfaction.

Basson's circular model provides a useful way of explaining to women that, although they may not feel spontaneous desire, if they are willing to be receptive to their partner, feelings of responsive desire may occur at or very near the time when arousal occurs. The rewards for women may be sexual satisfaction or feelings of closeness to their partner and pleasure in his or her sexual satisfaction. These feelings then increase women's willingness to be receptive on future occasions.

Another way of understanding responsive versus spontaneous desire is described by *Emily Nagoski*. Nagoski[5] suggests that desire is governed by accelerators and brakes. Accelerators are "turn-ons" and brakes are "turnoffs." Everyone has different turn-ons and turnoffs, and these may differ depending on the context in the moment.

Finally, the *Katz–Dizon model*[6] of male sexuality after cancer presents a bio-psycho-social model that describes sexual function in the context of the man's sexual identity and life. In this model, societal messages influence how the man experiences and expresses his sexuality. Sex drive is culturally bound, and sexual performance is centered on the penis. Body image and treatment side effects influence sexual performance in multiple ways, often resulting in sexual problems. The man's partner plays a key role in his sexual behavior and potential sexual recovery. Their communication is vital to both their satisfaction and his sexual performance during and after cancer treatment.

HUMAN SEXUAL BEHAVIOR

Sexual scripts are the learned behaviors, feelings, and meanings that people associate with sexual behavior. This is the "what" people do when they are preparing for or involved in sexual activity. Each person has learned an individual set of thoughts and actions that dictates the who, how, what, when, and where related to sexual activity. People start to learn these scripts by observing their parents and the way they display affection for one another.

Societal norms and messages from peers further influence one's thinking and behavior. When people enter a sexual relationship, they tend to use the same script over and over because that script is reinforced by pleasurable encounters. When the individual or couple is challenged by an illness that temporarily or permanently alters their anatomy or physiology, some will not be able to adapt their sexual scripts or behaviors, and sexual activity may end as a result.

CONCLUSION

Sexuality for human beings is a complex phenomenon comprising anatomic, hormonal, and behavioral aspects. Different models exist to explain this aspect of life, and these differ in their theoretical underpinnings. These models have shaped people's understanding of human sexuality, and continue to guide therapy and research in human sexuality.

Why does this matter? Knowing the how and why of the workings of our body is an important first step in seeking help and finding solutions to problems secondary to cancer and its treatments. We are all sexual beings, even if we are not actually having sex with a partner or self-pleasuring (masturbating). Our sexuality contributes to our sense of self and, for many, is part of our quality of life. When cancer or its treatments have a negative impact on any aspect of our sexuality, our sense of self and quality of life may suffer. Being able to talk about this with a partner or health-care provider will hopefully lead to both their understanding of what we are going through as well as potentially finding answers or solutions for what is bothering us.

CHAPTER 2

"Who will want me when I look like this?"

Body Image Changes

This chapter covers body image, which can undergo one of the most significant changes after cancer treatment. Body image, the way we see our physical self and how we feel about it, influences sexuality and is almost universally affected by the cancer experience. Up to 31% of women treated for breast cancer with surgery report changes in body image.[1] There is little research on the impact of cancer treatment on body image in men, suggesting that an assumption exists that men have robust body image compared to women and so this is not measured to any degree.

In this chapter you will hear the stories of two people dealing with physical changes as a result of cancer treatment. One of them is a single gay man who is concerned that scars from his surgery will affect his ability to establish a new relationship. The other is a woman who sees herself as "damaged" and distances herself from her partner, who no longer shares a bedroom with her.

JAMES

The past year had been nothing short of a disaster for James, who is 59 years old and who was diagnosed with colorectal cancer a year ago. He tried not to dwell on the memories of the cancer diagnosis and treatment, but they popped into his brain nonetheless. The day before, when he was driving home, the memory of his first week after the surgery where they'd removed a chunk of his bowel made him stop his car blocks from his house and sit for 10 minutes, trying to get his breath under control. He hated thinking about the surgery, but the memories kept coming back. The pain, the smells, the sounds . . . some of them emanating from his own body! He had always taken care of himself—regular exercise, healthy weight, minimal alcohol in recent years—so the diagnosis of colorectal cancer had been shocking. He had started chemotherapy and radiation within a week of the diagnosis, followed by the surgery that had resulted in a colostomy bag on his abdomen for nine months. Now, a year later, they were going to remove the bag and that hopefully would be the end of it. But would it?

James had barely looked at himself in the mirror since he'd come home from the hospital. He had to look at the bag when he was emptying and changing it, but other than that, his body was a no-go zone. He knew he had lost weight; his clothes were loose, and his face had developed sharp angles. He could see his weight loss reflected in the alarm on the faces of the few friends he had allowed to visit; his housekeeper continually tried to get him to eat more, but he ignored her as much as he could. The second time she'd brought him cupcakes from the bakery round the corner, he'd thrown them in the garbage, right in front of her. He knew he'd hurt her feelings, but she wouldn't listen when he told her he was not hungry—and certainly not for cupcakes with garish yellow frosting.

The physical changes brought about by cancer treatment can be challenging. They are a vivid reminder of the cancer diagnosis and prevent you from denying the reality of the situation you're in. They are also a visible sign to others that you have cancer; this can be stigmatizing or a trigger for sympathy, which for some can feel like pity.

James spent most days alone now; he had retired from his work as a city administrator when he'd been diagnosed, assuming that he'd had not much longer to live, and so why waste his remaining time on a job that was stressful and gave him little pleasure? But now, a year later, he was still alive, the days were long, and the nights gave little relief from boredom. While he certainly felt better physically, and he looked forward to getting rid of the "poop pal," as he called the ostomy bag, he was lonely but couldn't find the enthusiasm, or maybe it was the courage, to resume any form of social life.

He had been alone since the early 1990s, when his partner, Simon, had died of AIDS. James hated thinking about those days when so many of his friends had died from that dreadful disease. He thought he would never find love again, or even companionship, and for the last 30 years he'd lived by himself, sustaining a series of short relationships that never felt like love. And now, who would possibly want to be with him?

The fear of being seen as unattractive and thus not being able to be part of a couple is common in cancer survivors who are single. Emphasizing how you look as the only factor in finding love is limiting and can lead to avoiding opportunities where starting a new relationship may be possible.

The day of the surgery to close the ostomy arrived faster than James had anticipated. When the surgeon had told him this operation was "easier," James had given a half smile. Easier for the surgeon maybe, but what about him? He was surprised though by how quickly he recovered from the surgery to close the ostomy. Sure, it took a while to figure out his new bowel patterns, but that was minor compared to the time it had taken to come to terms with the ostomy bag. Now that he was free of that, he felt maybe he could get out a bit more . . .

His first attempt at socializing was to accept an invitation for cocktail hour at his friend Andrew's apartment. They had known each other for decades, and Andrew had been his main support after Simon had died. He had also been the most sensitive of James's friends after his first surgery, never pushing him to go out but calling regularly, even when James had been rude on the phone or had not answered his calls. It seemed fitting that James had agreed to the invitation, but he made Andrew promise it would be a small gathering with no surprise potential dates for James to meet.

It can be difficult to socialize after months of avoiding social situations. When you show visible signs of being treated for cancer, for example significant weight loss, going to a social event can feel overwhelming.

Getting ready for the event was more challenging than James had anticipated. He had mostly been wearing sweatpants during the year of treatment—yes, even to the clinic for the chemotherapy treatments—and finding something suitable for a social occasion seemed almost impossible. The worst part came after he'd showered, and he caught a glimpse of himself in the full-length mirror behind the bathroom door . . . He had purposely not looked at himself in that mirror since his first surgery, and the image of his naked body was much worse than he'd imagined.

There was a long pink scar that ran down the middle of his now concave stomach, with a curve around his belly button. Alongside the scar were what looked like puncture wounds, presumably from the sutures. On the right-hand side was a horizontal scar where the ostomy bag used to be; this wound looked healed but was bright red. He almost canceled on cocktails right there and then.

Surgical scars fade with time, but their initial appearance can be quite alarming. Initially red, over weeks and months they turn pink and then, in white people, white. For people of color, surgical wounds may look pink to start and eventually become more like the rest of the skin. Some people risk an overgrowth of scar tissue, called "keloid formation," which may require further treatment to shrink the additional tissue.

James called Andrew, the start of tears in his eyes. "I can't . . . I don't . . ." he stammered when his friend answered.

"I'll be right over!" Andrew left his apartment despite still having to finish the preparation for the gathering.

He was at James's door within minutes as he lived close by and had run most of the way. He found James in his bedroom, wrapped in a towel, his hair beginning to dry.

"What can't or don't you want to do?"

James gestured to his stomach.

"Oh that—no one is going to undress you, James, unless you want them to!"

James hadn't looked up at his friend, but he could hear the smile in his voice.

"Come on, now. Let's find something for you to wear. And if we don't find something, I have lots of outfits for you to choose from. I am rather more, um, svelte, shall we say, than you ever were!"

James felt a retort coming to his lips but stopped himself from replying. It was true, Andrew had always been admiringly thinner than James, who was shorter and more thickset than his friend. Andrew's offer of something to wear had cheered him up, just a little.

He put on a pair of worn sweatpants that Andrew wrinkled his nose at.

"We do have to go shopping soon, my friend. We can't have you wearing those for much longer. What a disgrace and, yes, I do know what you've gone through, but still . . ."

While wearing comfortable clothes is important during recovery from surgery, this can become a habit that's difficult to break. Baggy clothes may hide weight loss or weight gain, but they do little to improve self-image. Wearing well-fitting clothes is a key part of looking and feeling less like a patient and more like your normal self.

True to his word, Andrew found the perfect outfit for James. He politely left the room while James got dressed, and when James opened the door again, he had a smile on his face. He had to admit it felt good to be wearing pants and a crisp striped shirt after months in baggy T-shirts and sweatpants.

Andrew was waiting outside the room. "Wow! You clean up good, my friend. Now, how about a shave?"

James felt his face. He had grown a fairly substantial beard in the weeks since his last surgery, mostly because he was too lazy to shave. He could feel his cheekbones and chin through the mostly gray beard. "I'm kinda afraid to . . . I'm not sure what I look like under this . . ."

"I can't imagine you'll look any worse than you do now," Andrew muttered softly, not intending for James to hear.

"I heard that! Okay, let's get this off, but I can't promise that I won't grow it again if I really do look awful."

James was shocked when he looked closely at his face as the razor slid with some resistance over his skin. His face was pale, and he looked much older than his 59 years. When he was done, and the area around the sink was cleaned up, he hesitantly opened the bathroom door.

Andrew was once again waiting for him, this time holding out an ice-cold martini for James.

Making even small attempts at self-care, such as shaving or getting a haircut, can make a big difference in how you feel.

The evening was better, much better, than James had imagined. Firstly, Andrew hadn't invited anyone who'd known James in the "before cancer" days. The guests were mostly Andrew's colleagues from the HR company where he worked, and they were friendly and made an effort to avoid work talk and to include James in their conversations. Secondly, they were all about the same age as James and Andrew, and they seemed to travel a lot, so they had interesting stories to tell.

Before he knew it, the party started to wind down. It had been two hours since he'd arrived, and James was exhausted. Andrew hadn't offered anything to eat other than some cheese and crackers, and for the first time in ages, James was hungry. But he was unsure if he should have something to eat in the company of strangers. He was unsure if cheese was a "safe food" for his digestion—and what if something weird happened, like uncontrolled diarrhea? The others were talking about going to get burgers and fries at a nearby diner, but James begged off.

"I'm really tired for some reason. I think I need to go to bed more than I need heartburn," he joked.

Before the others could try to persuade him to go with them, Andrew stepped in. "I'm going to walk with James to his place, and I'll catch up with you. Order me a cheeseburger and sweet potato fries and a beer!"

James and Andrew chatted on the short walk to James's apartment.

"Thanks for making me come over tonight." James's voice was light. "I had a really good time. Your friends are very nice."

"Yes, they're a decent bunch. I'm not sure why I haven't introduced you before. Now, while you are still basking in the glow of your triumphant return to socializing, how about you agree to come with us—me and the same group—to the beach this weekend?"

The beach! That meant swimsuits and bare chests!

"Uh, no!" James's response was louder than he'd intended. "Absolutely not. Those days are over for me!"

"C'mon, it'll be great!"

"Do you not understand how hard it was for me to come to your place tonight? Do you have any idea how terrifying it is for me to expose myself to the stares and the looks full of pity?" The mood, so light just a few minutes before, was now white hot with James's anger.

"I'm sorry, I didn't know." Andrew had his hands out toward his friend in a gesture of apology.

James moved back out of reach. Without thinking, he lifted up the shirt he was wearing, right there on the sidewalk. "Look at me! Is this what you want to see on a day at the beach? Is this what anyone would want to see? It's enough to make anyone feel sick!"

Before Andrew could say anything, James had almost sprinted the last few steps to his apartment building. The glass panes of the front door rattled as he pulled it open and disappeared inside.

Being sensitive to others' reactions to scars or other physical changes is very common. Even if no one actually does stare— and of course some people will, and some will even ask about them—survivors are often hyperaware of reactions. Children in particular may ask about scars, so you might find it helpful to have a ready response.

James was calmer the next morning, and he called Andrew to apologize for his outburst. "I really am sorry for yelling at you like that." His voice was contrite. "But you have no idea . . ."

"I guess I don't have an idea of what it's like for you. But you're still here, and you still have a life to live!"

"Some life," was James's response.

"Exactly! I won't let you continue like this! You've been through a lot this year, but it's time to engage in your life again. I may be speaking out of turn, but I want my old friend James back."

"There is no 'old' James, Andrew! He's gone. Those days are over. No one is going to want to be with me, like they did with the 'old' James! I'm going to be alone forever, and that is all there is."

James was sobbing now, and he threw his phone on the bed, where it lay on top of the clothes he'd worn the night before. He could hear Andrew's voice calling his name through the phone, but he ignored it.

About an hour later, Andrew called back. James considered not answering but thought better of it.

"Hi Andrew. It seems that all I do these days is apologize to you. I really am sorry for how I acted . . . but so much has changed for me, and I don't know who I am anymore."

"Apology accepted, and I'm sorry for giving you a lecture. I don't know what life is like for you. But I know that I miss you and want you back in my life. Our other friends do too. You don't have to come to the beach, or go anywhere else for that matter, but would you consider something?"

"Sure, but I won't make any promises."

"How about we ease you in—maybe a walk on the beach, early in the morning or later in the afternoon? And we don't even have to go to our usual beach where all our friends go. Or used to go. None of us is in the same shape as we were in our glory days."

James had to laugh at this. If he was being honest, he hadn't been anywhere near the shape he'd been in their so-called glory days for a long time, none of them had. They were all in their late 50s or early 60s, and the young guys, the ones who still went to the bars or wherever they went to meet other men these days, didn't even look at Andrew and James!

"And you don't even have to wear a swimsuit!" Andrew said this with a laugh, but to James, it was a potential solution.

If the fear of exposing yourself is keeping you from going out or participating in exercise or sports, consider wearing clothing that covers your scars or stretch marks. Going to the beach doesn't mean you have to wear a swimsuit; for different reasons, many people avoid the sun and wear some sort of covering to protect their skin, so you won't necessarily stand out.

It took a couple of weeks for James to find the courage, but on one of the last hot days of the summer, he called Andrew and invited him to go for a beach picnic, T-shirts required.

LETITIA AND ROGER

Letitia is a 48-year-old woman who was diagnosed with breast cancer two months ago. Her husband, Roger, has been with her every step of the way from the moment she returned from the doctor's office where she'd heard the dreaded words "You have cancer."

She didn't say anything as she took off her jacket; she didn't need to. He looked at her face and put his arms around her and didn't let go until she moved away from him.

"It's going to be okay, honey," was all he said. And, in the early days after the surgery, that was what he said every time she encountered a challenge or cried with frustration when she couldn't find the energy to go for a walk. She'd had surgery to remove her breast and immediate reconstruction, something that she thought was going to have the least impact on her body image and that was recommended by the surgeon.

While Roger wasn't used to cooking, he tried his best to make most of their meals—until Letitia begged him to give up and let her sister, Lorena, bring them meals. He could warm up soup from a can and make fried eggs, but he often burned the toast. Soup or eggs and toast lost their appeal after a week or two, but by the third week after her surgery, Letitia was able to warm up a casserole or boil pasta.

In the immediate period after she'd come home from the hospital, Roger had slept in the spare room so as not to disturb her. He missed her at night, her soft snoring lulling him to sleep and her warm body lying close to him in the cool nights. But it was now two months later, and there had been no move by either of them for him to return to their bed. Roger was not sure why he was still in the spare room, and he waited patiently for Letitia to raise the topic, but she said nothing.

It took him a while to notice that other things had changed too; she closed the bedroom door when she got ready for bed, and in the morning, she appeared fully clothed when she came to the kitchen to make coffee. This was unusual, but he kept quiet because he didn't want to upset her. She had been moody ever since the diagnosis, and while he understood why and was patient, he wished she would return soon to the Letitia who was easygoing and almost always in a good mood. She had also stopped going for her daily walks, and he wondered if this was part of her grumpiness.

Letitia shared some of her feelings with her twin sister, Lorena. They were extremely close, something that had bothered Roger when he and Letitia had first started dating, but after 20 years together, he had become used to it. The sisters shared almost everything, and Lorena almost always knew what Letitia was feeling before she shared it with Roger. Lorena was a nurse, so Roger wasn't surprised that his wife turned to her twin for advice on anything health related.

Letitia had talked with Lorena about how she was frustrated at how long it was taking her to feel like herself again. She was worried about why her reconstructed breast was misshapen, and she wondered whether perhaps her surgery had been messed up in some way.

"Can you show me what you mean?" asked Lorena.

"Well, okay, but honestly I have hardly looked myself . . ." Letitia hesitated before slowly opening her shirt.

"Hmmm," Lorena said. "Remember, I'm not a surgical nurse, but that looks normal to me."

Letitia immediately turned from her sister and buttoned up her shirt again.

It can take months for the swelling from breast reconstruction surgery to subside, and the absence of one or both breasts alters how clothes fit or look. This can come as a shock and cause distress. Women often avoid looking at themselves undressed as a coping mechanism, and the sight of their altered body can be upsetting.

Letitia's recovery was slow but steady, and after another month, she felt well enough to go back to work at the nonprofit organization where she was the volunteer coordinator. This was when she encountered another hurdle. None of her work clothes fit properly! She had not looked at her breasts since the dressings had come off. On the weekend before she went back to the office, she went through her closet to get organized for the week ahead. Within minutes she was in tears; she sat on her bed, shirts and blouses strewn all around her. What was she going to do?

Her sister came to the rescue as she had so many times before. Lorena brought over a pile of loose-fitting tops and a couple of athletic bras that, while not attractive or anything resembling the lacy bras Letitia favored, at least fit. With Lorena's gentle encouragement, Letitia looked at herself in the mirror. Her two breasts looked different, and this brought on the tears again. Her "new" reconstructed breast was a different shape from her "normal" breast, and there was a reddish scar that ran horizontally across it. Her nipple and surrounding tissue were gone as well!

"Take a few deep breaths, L." Her sister's nursing training was on full display. "It's always a shock when you first see the scar, but that will change. And the important thing is that the cancer is gone, right?"

Letitia nodded—that was the most important thing—but still . . . what she saw in the mirror upset her more than she'd been prepared for. She was grateful she didn't need any additional treatment such as chemotherapy or radiation. But she and Roger were still sleeping in separate rooms, almost three months after her surgery. She dressed and undressed in the bathroom or in the bedroom with the door firmly closed. Once he'd walked into the bedroom when she'd been standing in her underwear, and her response startled him—she'd gasped and raced into the en suite bathroom, slamming the door behind her. After that, he'd made sure to knock loudly or avoid entering the bedroom at all when she was in there with the door closed.

It's not unusual for women to hide all or part of their physical appearance after breast cancer surgery. Some women report feeling that they've been mutilated by removal of the breast, even with reconstructive surgery.

Roger hadn't said anything or asked why this had continued, and the space between them grew wider every day. Neither of them seemed willing to break the silence, and they were now living like college roommates. Roger's unhappiness was visible to Lorena when she came to visit, but she too kept silent and didn't ask her sister about what was going on.

But one night, Roger spoke up.

"Letitia, I can't take it anymore! What is going on with you? With us? It's like we're strangers under this roof! I don't know what to do anymore!"

Letitia was shocked by the pain in his voice. She recognized the way they were living was not normal or making either of them happy, but she didn't know how to narrow the distance between them. She looked at her husband, tears in her eyes. "I . . . I don't know what to say! I'm sorry, that's all I know . . . so sorry . . ." Now she was crying, her hands over her face, as if hiding her tears would somehow stop them.

Roger always felt helpless when she cried, but now that he'd started talking, he couldn't stop. "I thought, I hoped that by now things would be back to normal between us! But you're even further away from me, if that's even possible! I am so lonely."

Now *he* was crying, and that stopped Letitia's tears; she had never seen him cry, not in all 20 years of their relationship. She turned and put her arms around him, hugging him tight. It was the first time they had been this close physically since the night before her surgery. After a couple of minutes, she pulled away from him, blew her nose, and offered him a tissue. They both sat down on the couch, a space between them.

"Please talk to me." Roger's voice was soft. "I don't know what you're going through, and I can't help you . . . if you even want my help!"

"I don't know what I need or want! It's too much, all of this!"

"What is too much?" Roger was desperate to understand what she was going through. "Would it help if you spoke to someone? Like a professional?"

"What is that going to do?" Letitia was immediately defensive.

"Is there someone that Lorena may know? She's connected at the hospital to all sorts of people. Maybe one of her nursing friends . . . Can you ask her?"

Before she spoke, Letitia looked at Roger. She could see how upset he was, and if she were honest with herself, she was more unhappy than she'd ever been.

"Okay, I'll ask Lorena. I promise."

It was almost as if Lorena had been waiting for her to ask for help. She had three suggestions of people Letitia could talk to, starting off with one of her nurse friends who worked at the cancer center. Because Letitia hadn't needed chemotherapy after the mastectomy, she hadn't been referred there, but her sister assured her that she could still contact her nursing colleague. This woman's name was Brenda, and before she lost her nerve, Letitia called and left a message for her.

Brenda called back within the hour. She explained to Letitia that she was something called a "nurse navigator," and that if Letitia answered a few questions, Brenda could help her find someone to assist her further.

Nurse navigators are specially trained registered nurses who work in most major cancer centers. Their role is to help patients and survivors navigate the system and get connected to the services they need. Navigators are usually attached to departments that either treat specific types of cancer or provide specific types of treatments.

Letitia hesitated before speaking. "I don't know if this is something you deal with, but well, I had breast cancer, and I had surgery and reconstruction—" Letitia felt her throat tighten up, but she forced herself to keep talking. "It's just that I know I'm lucky that I didn't need chemo or any other treatment but . . ." She took a deep breath, and the words spilled out of her.

She told Brenda how she hated her body now, and none of her clothes fit properly, and she had to wear clothes that she hated, and she didn't want to go out, and it was affecting her marriage. She barely stopped talking once she'd started; Brenda listened and did not interrupt. Finally, Letitia stopped, and there was a short silence.

"Thank you for sharing that," Brenda said softly but clearly. "This is something I see quite frequently. If you're interested, we can set up an appointment for you to see me here at the cancer center, and if I can't help you, I can refer you to someone in our psychology department."

"Oh, thank you!" Letitia felt comfortable with the nurse, after only their brief conversation, and she'd told her everything. She did not want to have to repeat herself to someone else.

They set up an appointment for early the next week. The nurse navigator started work early in the morning, so Letitia could see her and get to work on time. Letitia felt nervous as she drove to the appointment; she saw herself as someone who could handle most situations, but here she was, seeking help from a stranger, for the first time in her life.

"Let me start off by telling you again that many women struggle with the physical changes after breast cancer surgery. This is not something you can prepare yourself for, and you've made an important first step in helping yourself overcome or at least come to terms with the changes."

Letitia found herself relaxing as Brenda spoke.

"You're just over two months away from a life-changing event, so cut yourself some slack! Not only is your body settling into its new form but so is your brain! Now let me suggest some practical strategies to help you with this new reality."

Brenda told Letitia the scars would fade with time, but they would never go away. She asked Letitia whether the absence of the nipple and areola on her affected breast bothered her; Letitia had not thought about that, and in that moment, she realized it did bother her. Brenda told her she could have the areola tattooed on and a nipple surgically created. Why had no one told her about that, Letitia wondered. Brenda said that until Letitia was comfortable looking at her "new" breast in the mirror, she should not beat herself up about avoiding her husband, but she did need to tell him what she was going through.

"I don't know if I will ever be okay about him seeing this." Letitia gestured toward her breasts.

Brenda nodded. "I'm not a sex therapist, but you don't have to be naked or have your breasts exposed—or touched—if you're not comfortable or if it makes you anxious or upset," Brenda explained. "If wearing something that covers your breast or both breasts helps you to relax and be present in the moment, that's okay. But you need to talk to your husband about your feelings. I know I'm repeating myself about talking to him, but that's more important than anything else at this stage."

Letitia sighed. She knew she needed to talk to Roger, but why was it so difficult?

When it comes to something that's difficult to talk about, you might find it easier to talk to a professional, or even a stranger, than to someone you love. The "emotional temperature" isn't as high, and there is no risk of hurting the person's feelings.

"And as for the clothing issue," Brenda continued, "wearing clothes that you're not comfortable in and that make you feel unattractive may just make you feel worse. While your body is adjusting, finding a couple of outfits that make you feel good might help. Trying to make your 'before' clothes work for you tends to highlight what has changed."

That made a lot of sense to Letitia. In fact, Brenda had given her a lot of good advice, and she was grateful.

"I really do need to get to work." Letitia started to get up from the chair. "Can I contact you again if I need to?"

"Of course," Brenda replied as she rose from her chair. "Here is a list of support groups that you might find useful. The women who attend are going through the same stuff as you are, and they can share what worked for them and what didn't. They also know about other resources you can access. I also have a list of couple therapists if you think that you and your husband may need some help talking."

Letitia drove to work with so many thoughts whirling in her head. She did need to buy some new clothes, and maybe she would try a support group, but one thing she knew for sure—she needed to talk to Roger, first and foremost.

That night, Letitia told Roger about her appointment with the nurse navigator. She recounted the advice she'd gotten about joining a support group and buying some new clothes, and about the need to talk to him about how she was feeling. As she talked, she could see the worry on his face ease. She also felt her own frustration and sadness begin to lift. She realized this conversation was just a start, and she still had work to do. But it was a start—a good start.

CONCLUSION

Body image is an important aspect of how people see themselves in relation to their sexual self-image. It's not possible to prepare for all the potential changes after cancer treatment. The physical changes after surgery, radiation, or chemotherapy all affect body image, and some of these changes may be permanent. As a result, you might hide the changes from your partner by undressing and dressing behind closed doors. It can also be difficult to talk to anyone about your feelings related to the changes. But talking about the changes, and your associated feelings, is an important step in accepting the reality and moving on.

TAKEAWAYS

- Any surgery can alter body image and one's sense of self. Body image is highly influenced by society; trends in what is attractive come and go.

- Changes to the body as a result of cancer treatment are often not talked about openly. Distress with the changes is not unique to women, as is often thought; men experience this too.

- There is no quick fix for the emotional response to the physical changes, but acknowledging your feelings about this is the first step in coming to terms with these changes.

- Seeking help from a professional or others who've had a similar experience can help lessen feelings of isolation or that there's no help for your situation.

- Buying a few items of clothing that fit and make you feel good, rather than trying to wear ill-fitting clothes, can also help. Your body will change over time after surgery, so even just one or two new items at a time can be a morale boost.

- If you can't afford a completely new wardrobe, borrowing from family or friends (they will be happy to help!) or shopping at a secondhand store may be a good solution.

WEBSITES FOR ADDITIONAL INFORMATION

Breastcancer.org (an education and support service for people with breast cancer)

https://www.breastcancer.org/managing-life/taking
-care-of-mental-health/body-image

CancerCare
https://www.cancercare.org/tagged/body_image

Macmillan Cancer Support (United Kingdom)
https://www.macmillan.org.uk/cancer-information
-and-support/impacts-of-cancer/changes-to-your
-appearance-and-body-image

National Cancer Institute (NIH)
https://www.cancer.gov/about-cancer/coping/self
-image

CHAPTER 3

"I have no interest in sex—will it ever come back?"

Absence of Desire

Libido, or sexual desire, can be affected by a range of cancer treatments and is often an emotional response to the entire cancer experience. Androgen deprivation therapy for men with recurrent or advanced prostate cancer is a mainstay of treatment, and profound loss of libido is a common side effect for 64% of men receiving this treatment.[1] For women, loss of desire is common when being treated for cancer; this occurs in up to 87% of women[2] and is associated with body image changes as well as sexual pain[3] or loss of sexual function. Relationship conflict is another factor contributing to loss of libido. This chapter describes the experiences of two couples where loss of sexual desire as a result of a cancer diagnosis or treatment is having an impact on their relationship.

BRIAN AND SANDRA

Brian and Sandra have been married for 15 years; this is a second marriage for both of them. Brian's wife died 3 years before he met Sandra, and she had been divorced for almost a decade when she met Brian. They are both in their mid-60s and retired one year apart, with Brian leaving his position as a bank manager before Sandra, who had owned a children's clothing store, also retired. Their plan was to travel extensively during their retirement years; neither of them have children, so they have no obligations other than an elderly cat, whom they board with a neighbor.

Their plans fell apart when Brian was diagnosed with an aggressive form of prostate cancer one year ago. He was offered radiation therapy with two years of androgen deprivation therapy. Sandra didn't understand why he didn't have his prostate removed; this made more sense to her than leaving the offending organ in his body, but Brian told her these therapies were recommended by the doctors at the cancer center, and who was he to argue with the experts? Brian and Sandra were supposed to be in Mexico for four of the six weeks of treatment, and he was annoyed they'd had to cancel their trip. But the radiation therapy went smoothly, even though he was increasingly fatigued as the weeks went by.

When he started the radiation therapy, he also started a course of androgen deprivation therapy. Neither Brian nor Sandra had ever heard this term before, and when she looked online, Sandra read that the medication would stop Brian's body from producing testosterone. There was a long list of side effects that sounded scary, but Brian reassured her that the doctor had told him the medication was well tolerated and he would be "fine." For Brian, that was enough to tell Sandra she shouldn't worry.

Androgen deprivation therapy, often called "hormone therapy," has global side effects on a man's body. The term "hormone therapy" is inaccurate in this case; it suggests the medication is providing additional hormones, while it is in fact doing the opposite—stopping production of the male hormone testosterone.

But Sandra did worry. As the weeks went by, even after his radiation therapy was over, Brian became more irritable and fatigued. They had expected he would be tired while undergoing the radiation, but they had been assured this would get better with time. In fact, it was getting worse and wasn't relieved even when he took a long afternoon nap. The problem wasn't just a matter of needing long naps; he had no energy and didn't want to do anything other than sit in his chair, watching television. And his irritability was causing them to argue, something they'd rarely done before his diagnosis.

It seemed to Sandra as if nothing she did were right. The toast was too dark and the soup not hot enough. He flew off the handle when he couldn't find the shirt he'd worn the previous day, as if this were her fault. But he'd forgotten he'd thrown it in the laundry basket after he'd spilled ketchup on it the night before. These small things wouldn't have bothered him in the "before" days, but now they were the trigger for an argument. It didn't take Sandra long to start to watch her words, especially if she disagreed with him. Speaking up just wasn't worth the fight that would ensue, but these changes made her wonder what was happening to him—and to them as a consequence. She once again searched the internet for information about the side effects of his medication. She read every word, and what she saw confirmed some of the changes her husband was showing. The list was long—irritability, fatigue and loss of energy, weight gain, memory loss, loss of upper-body muscle mass, and sexual dysfunction. The last item on the list made her sit back in the chair, her brow creased. When was the last time they'd had sex? Now that she thought about it, when was the last time they'd even kissed or hugged?

Most men on androgen deprivation therapy experience a range of sexual problems, including loss of desire, erectile difficulties, and shrinkage of the penis and scrotum.

Sandra could not remember when they'd last had sex. Sure, things had cooled down after the first year or two of their relationship, but an absence this long was unusual. They'd avoided having sex while Brian was going through the radiation, but they hadn't talked about any reason to abstain, and the doctor hadn't mentioned any. Sandra assumed it had something to do with exposing her to radiation, but she wasn't sure. They'd still hugged and kissed good night, but then that had stopped at some point too, she just couldn't remember when. She decided she would ask Brian after dinner that night whether he knew what was going on with them.

Couples often worry that if they have sex, or even kiss, while one of them is undergoing radiation therapy, the partner can be exposed to the radiation. This is not true; the radiation is not "passed" to the partner. But radiation to the pelvic area can cause skin or tissue damage, and sexual intercourse may further damage the tissues and increase the risk of infection.

Brian's reaction to what Sandra regarded as a carefully worded question was extreme in her opinion.

"What do you mean?" He was almost yelling. "I don't know what you're talking about!"

"Brian, honey . . ." Sandra tried to keep her voice calm. "We haven't kissed or hugged for ages. Is there something that I've done? Or have you found someone else?"

He didn't answer and stormed away from the table, leaving the dishes rattling.

Sandra sat there, confused and upset. What had she said to cause such a reaction? The longer she sat, the more her thoughts raced. Could he be having an affair? That had to be the only reason for such an overreaction! She tried to think of any behavior of his that would support what she would normally think of as absurd. She'd never had any reason to not trust him before, not once in the 15 years of their marriage. He knew her first husband had cheated on her more than once and how soul destroying that had been for her. And it wasn't as if Brian were sneaking around; in fact, he was home more than he'd ever been. So why was he so angry with her question?

Partners of men on androgen deprivation therapy may confuse the man's loss of desire as evidence of cheating. Or they may misinterpret the man's withdrawal or lack of interest to be a result of something they themself might have done. The man may react to a question about his behavior as if it were an accusation. If the couple doesn't talk about these concerns openly, misunderstandings will continue and even increase.

The distance between them continued to grow. Sandra searched the internet for more information and found a website for the spouses of men with advanced prostate cancer. One of the articles she read told the story of a couple where, like Brian, the man was on androgen deprivation therapy, and his spouse described a change in their relationship almost identical to what she and Brian were experiencing. The woman in the article was convinced the man's lack of interest in her was a result of her gaining weight because of the stress of his diagnosis and treatment. Sandra felt like laughing at this; she had *lost* weight since Brian's diagnosis! But the lesson for her from the story was that the man's lack of interest had nothing to do with the woman and everything to do with the loss of testosterone. The article concluded with a description of how the couple went to see a sex therapist and resolved their problem. Sandra wondered, would this work for her and Brian?

Sandra's next step was to try and find a sex therapist in their city. She found contact information for a number of therapists, but she was not sure exactly what services they provided. A couple of them had what looked like psychology degrees, and some were social workers. Just two of them had certification as a sex therapist, and she called the first one on her list. A woman with a friendly voice answered the phone, and they had a brief conversation, at the end of which Sandra had an appointment in two weeks . . . but how was she going to tell Brian about this?

There are a variety of professionals who can be consulted for help when a couple is experiencing sexual problems. Asking a trusted friend or primary care provider for a recommendation may be useful, but that means acknowledging to another person that there is a problem in your relationship, and this isn't always easy to do. It's important to understand the difference between different kinds of professionals, and checking their professional credentials is vital. You may also need to see more than one counsellor before you find someone who is "right" for both you and your partner.

The opportunity for Sandra to talk to Brian presented itself about a week later. They were watching television, and Sandra sat down next to Brian on the couch. He immediately got up and moved to a chair.

"Why did you move?" Sandra couldn't hide the hurt in her voice.

"Because I know what you are doing, and I don't like it!" was his reply.

"What am I doing?"

"You're . . . It's plain to see . . . You know darn well what you're trying to do!"

"I sat down next to you! Is that a crime?" Sandra's voice was getting louder.

"I know what you want, and you can't have it, and you need help!"

Here was her chance to tell him about the appointment with the therapist.

"*We* need help, Brian! And I've made an appointment for us to get that help!"

The words were out, and they stopped Brian from saying anything else. Sandra was silent as she waited for him to respond.

After what seemed like hours but was just a few seconds, he spoke. "What do you mean?" His voice was quiet. "What have you done? What appointment?"

Sandra told him about the appointment with the sex therapist, except she left out the "sex" part. She told him the changes in their relationship, the distance that had grown between them, were making her so unhappy that in desperation she had contacted a professional to help them with whatever had gone wrong since he'd started treatment.

Brian grunted in response. But he had to admit things hadn't been right between them for a while. He didn't know why, but he sure wasn't happy, and it seemed neither was his wife. "Okay, okay. We'll go to this therapist person, but I'm not promising anything."

The day of the appointment arrived, and until they were at the therapist's office building, Sandra wasn't sure Brian would attend. He was quiet on the drive there, and he walked slowly toward the entrance, a worried look on his face. Sandra ignored this behavior but waited for him to enter the elevator with her. Then, at the end of a long corridor, Sandra firmly knocked on the therapist's door. It was opened by a short woman with curly red hair that sprung out of a loose bun on the top of her head.

"Sandra? Good morning and welcome. I'm Dr. Shepherd, but you can call me Amanda. And this must be your partner." The woman held out her hand toward Brian, who shook it quickly and then put his hand in his pocket. "Come on in. I sit there," she said, pointing to a leather chair. "You can both sit on the couch, or if you wish, I can pull up another chair next to the couch."

"We can sit on the couch," replied Sandra as she sat down and gestured for Brian to sit next to her.

"Let me tell you a little about what I do."

Dr. Shepherd—Amanda—explained that she was a sex therapist, and Sandra felt Brian stiffen, his eyes boring into the side of her head, but she didn't look at him. The therapist continued to say that she helped couples who were experiencing not just sexual problems but also communication barriers and other relationship challenges. Each time she said the word "sexual" or "sex," Sandra's breath caught in her throat as she imagined Brian's face.

"So why don't we start with either one of you telling me why you are here today."

Sandra looked at Brian, who was gazing at the art on the walls. She took a deep breath, and the words tumbled out of her. She was looking at the therapist as she spoke and didn't notice the look on Brian's face. She described how distant they had become and how he avoided any physical contact with her. She said she thought it had something to do with the medication he was on, and she had read that this was possible, but she was afraid to talk to Brian about it. She described how he'd gotten angry with her when she'd tried to touch him. When she eventually stopped talking, she looked at Brian and was surprised to see he had tears in his eyes.

"Brian, if I may call you that," Dr. Shepherd said softly, "what are you thinking?"

"I—I had no idea," he stammered. "Sandra, why didn't you tell me?"

"I did tell you! I told you, and you denied that anything had changed between us! I miss you! I miss us!" Sandra looked at the therapist. "Dr. Shepherd, have you seen other couples where this is happening? Can you help us?"

The doctor cleared her throat and then spoke with authority in her voice. "The short answer is that a lot of what you describe is a side effect of the testosterone-blocking medication. And yes, I have seen this before. I've worked with other couples where the man has been treated for prostate cancer, and the impact on the couple is significant. But there is more to this than just the loss of testosterone."

Brian finally spoke. His voice was shaky, but there was also an element of relief in his words. If this was a side effect of the medication, he said, then they could just wait it out, couldn't they?

"But what do we do in the meantime?" Sandra was not satisfied with his wait-and-see response. He was supposed to be on this medication for two years, and they were just halfway through; she dreaded the thought of another 12 months of the fighting and distance between them.

"There are likely a range of behaviors and misunderstandings that have created the situation you're in now." Dr. Shepherd's voice was firm. "Underlying the irritability and other mood changes are the changes in masculinity that most men experience. The loss of sexual desire and sexual function is a major part of this, but so is the increased sensitivity and loss of what I call 'vim and vigor.' Does this make sense to you, Brian?"

He could only nod as he fought the tears that were about to flood his eyes. Sandra reached out to hold his hand, and he instinctively pulled away.

"See, Dr. Shepherd, did you see what he just did? That's what happens every time I try to touch him!"

It's not uncommon for couples to actively avoid touching each other when libido has changed. This stems from a combination of past behavior (touch = initiation of something sexual) and lack of communication (sometimes a hug is just a hug and not an invitation for or a precursor to sexual activity).

"How did that make you feel, Sandra?"

"It hurts to be rejected like that. I was trying to show him that I care about him, and it's not all, or even a little bit, about sex. I love him, and I hate to see him suffering like this . . ."

"And Brian, do you hear what Sandra is saying?"

"I guess so," Brian mumbled. "Maybe I haven't looked at things from her perspective. But what can I—what can we—do about this mess we've gotten into?"

"Ah!" said the therapist with the beginnings of a smile on her face. "That is where I can help you. It's about communication firstly, and about mutual understanding, and then about touch, and maybe we'll eventually get to the sex part . . . if you're will-ing to stick with therapy for a bit. What do you say?"

Brian and Sandra nodded in unison, and this time it was Brian who reached out to hold his spouse's hand.

COLLEEN AND JEREMY

Colleen and Jeremy are both 27 years old and were married a couple of years ago. They had known each other since their col-lege days but connected romantically only when he moved into the same apartment complex as Colleen. Theirs is a com-fortable relationship with common interests (theater, cocktails, and hiking), and they have a large social group. They both work as graphic designers but in competing firms, which makes for little work talk owing to concerns about confidentiality.

Colleen had been diagnosed with cervical cancer six months after their wedding. She'd had a couple of concerning Pap tests in the years before that, but the progression to an aggressive form of the cancer had alarmed her doctors and scared her to the core. Jeremy had been her primary support through the months of treatment, and he'd insisted on taking a leave of ab-sence from work so that he could care for her.

It had taken Colleen months to start feeling like herself after the initial surgery followed by radiation therapy and chemo-therapy. She experienced pretty much every side effect possible from the various treatments. She had a severe infection after the surgery that delayed the start of the radiation. Then she suffered extensive radiation burns that made sitting or standing ex-tremely painful. And the chemotherapy she was given caused significant nausea and vomiting that was difficult to control. It was as if anything that could go wrong did.

Colleen had finally gone back to work three months ago, and their social life, while nowhere near what it used to be, was getting busier. She'd lost almost 30 pounds during treatment and was slowly gaining the weight back, but it wasn't easy. Her work colleagues brought her muffins and cupcakes on a regular basis, and while she was grateful, she preferred to eat protein and fresh fruits and vegetables to regain muscle mass. Earning a salary again was also a relief for both of them; they'd had to dip into their savings during the many months she couldn't work.

Colleen attended the survivorship program at the cancer center where she'd been treated. It was a comprehensive program, and while she didn't see an oncologist at every visit, she was happy to see the nurse practitioner who ran the program. Her name was Marcy, and she was a couple of years older than Colleen. She was easy to talk to and didn't seem rushed, as opposed to many of the oncologists who tended to speed through her post-treatment appointments.

At one appointment, after talking about how she was feeling and taking her vital signs, Marcy asked Colleen a question that took her completely by surprise. "How are things between you and Jeremy these days?"

It was a simple question, but Colleen didn't know what to say. No one had asked her how they were doing as a couple in all the months of treatment, not her friends or family members, and not anyone on her cancer team. She wasn't sure how many of Jeremy's friends had asked him how he was doing, or if anyone at all had asked. Of course, he may not have told them about her cancer and treatments, but he hadn't said anything to her about any conversations.

Now here was the nurse practitioner asking her how *they* were doing, and she didn't have a good answer.

"Um, fine, I guess . . ." was the best she could manage.

But things were not fine.

Marcy wasn't satisfied with Colleen's half-hearted response. "What does 'fine' mean?" Her voice was soft, but the question got through to Colleen.

"I guess . . . it's . . . well, I'm not sure how okay we are. Things are just . . . um . . . different between us since the cancer. It's been just over 18 months, and we seem—just 'distant' is the best way I can describe it." Her voice was shaky as she admitted to Marcy what she had not really admitted even to herself.

The reality was that she and Jeremy really were distant from each other. They talked about social plans or what needed to be done around their apartment, but they hadn't really talked about anything substantial for a long time; conversations had become mostly transactional. Jeremy regularly asked her how she was feeling, and every time she said she was fine, and he didn't ask anything further.

It's common for couples to avoid "deep" conversations when they're struggling to keep their heads above water with the daily challenges of work and household tasks. They may be wary of bringing up sensitive or painful topics, and so they just coast, their interactions superficial.

Additionally, they hadn't had sex since before her treatment, other than the one time they'd tried but had to stop because it was painful for Colleen. She'd pushed Jeremy away and then started crying. When she'd looked at his face, she saw that he didn't understand what had happened. She'd explained to him that it had hurt, really hurt, and then he'd started to cry because he'd caused her pain. She hated to see him cry, and she'd ended up comforting him when she was the one who'd needed comforting! All of that had happened soon after she'd completed radiation therapy, and it was the last time they'd even tried to have sex. Even though she wanted to talk to him about this, it was difficult for her to raise the topic. Because she had a gynecologic cancer, she had assumed she might have some side effects from the treatment, but no one had said anything to her other than she should not have sex for six weeks after surgery. And then the radiation therapy had caused burns to her buttocks, lower abdomen, and genitals. Jeremy had been understanding during that time, and since then as well. And so sex had fallen off her radar, and anyway, she was always so tired after work . . .

It was clear to Marcy that Colleen was having difficulty talking about her relationship, so she decided to be more forthright in how she approached the topic. "How are things going for *you*? The note from the gynecological oncologist you saw states that you were not fully healed after the radiation."

Colleen's face told Marcy what she needed to know—her patient was not all that "fine." But Marcy pressed on. "Women often have a difficult time with sex after treatment," she said. "And it's often not easy to talk about. But problems with sex often lead to relationship problems too."

Colleen wasn't looking at the nurse; she was looking at her hands, which were twisting a sodden tissue. Colleen hadn't made a sound, but Marcy could see tears dripping down her cheeks. Marcy pushed the box of tissues closer to the young woman and sat quietly, waiting for her to stop crying or at least gain some composure.

"I think . . . it seems . . . I mean . . . I think our sex life is over!" She was now sobbing. "It's been I don't know how many months, more than a year at least, and I'm scared that Jeremy isn't going to be able to wait anymore for me to be, well, normal!"

"Okay, I hear you, but take a deep breath, and let's start at the beginning."

With some gentle prompting from Marcy, Colleen was able to describe what had happened over the previous months. She told the nurse about the one occasion when they had tried to have sex and how painful it was. She assured Marcy that Jeremy had been patient, but she knew his patience was wearing thin. She told the nurse that, beyond her fear that sex would always be painful, she was sure something was broken inside her because she never wanted to have sex, and she never used to be this way.

"Okay, thanks for telling me that," Marcy said. "Can we talk some more about this? I have a few questions that should help me perhaps help you."

Colleen nodded. Now that she had told Marcy some of what she was feeling, maybe the nurse could provide some advice.

"Let me make sure I understand what you've told me," the nurse continued. "It sounds to me like there are a couple issues going on here. First, you tried to have sex, and it really hurt. And now you have no desire for sex. Have I got that right?"

It sounded so simple when Marcy put it like that. But it was not simple, thought Colleen.

Marcy seemed to read her mind. "It's not simple at all," she said.

Pain with sex—not just with vaginal penetration but with sexual touch of any kind—is often the cause of a lack of interest or desire. This is a natural and normal response; why be interested in something that's painful?

"If sex hurts, why would you want it? But let me ask something. Can you tell me what things were like before your diagnosis?" The nurse asked the question gently.

"Do you mean when we first got together, Jeremy and I?"

Marcy laughed quietly. "Don't we all wish things remained like they were in the beginning?"

Even Colleen laughed. "Yeah, those were the days . . . No, of course things weren't like that for very long. But I still wanted him, you know? And now, there's nothing. I never feel like it, it never even occurs to me . . . so then we don't even try. What's wrong with me?"

"There's nothing wrong with you, Colleen. You are responding in a completely normal way to what has happened to you. But there may be something I can explain that might help."

Women often assume that for sex to happen they have to want it. In other words, they assume that desire, or sexual interest, has to be there before sex can happen. For many men, there is a linear process involved; desire, arousal, sexual activity, then orgasm, in that order. It is different for many women, where desire happens at the same time as arousal. So, if a woman waits for her interest or desire to happen, and it doesn't, she then thinks and acts as if sex is not going to happen.

As Marcy explained this, Colleen found herself with more questions. "Are you saying that I should have sex even if I don't want to?"

Marcy shook her head. "Not entirely. You should not do anything you don't want to do. But there's a difference between not wanting to do something and not having spontaneous desire for sex. It's unlikely that, after years of being together, things are going to be the same as they were in the early days of a relationship, when you could hardly wait to get your hands on your partner."

"Okay, I get that, but what can I do?" Colleen was getting a little frustrated with the way the conversation was going. Now that she had admitted to Marcy that things in her relationship were not "fine," she wanted to fix them.

The nurse took a deep breath. "We need to talk about the pain, but more generally, if you have no spontaneous desire initially, that doesn't mean you won't feel desire when you experience arousal." Marcy explained that for many women, desire is responsive rather than spontaneous. Desire happens when a woman is aroused rather than as a feeling that occurs randomly or when a woman sees her partner.

Many women identify with the idea that desire is responsive rather than spontaneous. The idea also provides hope that desire is possible. If the couple get something started—maybe a massage or some kissing and cuddling—that's when desire happens, in response to touch. The partner may get aroused, but the couple should discuss what to do about that beforehand. If the woman is still not interested, and her partner is aroused, the partner may want to masturbate or take a cold shower. What is important is that communication takes place and that the couple are prepared for what might happen.

"We do still need to talk about the pain you experienced in the past and what might help, but in the meanwhile, how about you talk to Jeremy about what we talked about today, and see if he's willing to try and see if you experience responsive desire with some, um, encouragement in the form of fooling around?"

"Okay," Colleen said, "but what happens if by some miracle I do find that I want to have sex?"

Marcy was a little surprised that Colleen seemed so eager to try; she'd thought she might be more cautious. "Well, if that happens, make sure you have some lube available and take it easy. I'm not going to tell you that you can't have sex, but there is a chance that if you have pain again, it might set you back. You may need to see a pelvic floor physiotherapist if the pain persists."

Colleen's face reflected the realization that this was not going to be a quick fix.

They agreed to make another appointment for the following week, after Colleen talked with Jeremy.

That night after dinner as they were cleaning up the kitchen, Jeremy asked Colleen how her appointment had gone. She hesitated for a moment. Was this a good time to talk to him? But it was the perfect segue . . .

"It was good. You remember Marcy? The nurse practitioner that I really like? Well, we spent a long time talking about something that you and I should really talk about . . ."

Jeremy looked up from the dish he was drying. This sounded serious, so he put down the plate and dish towel and leaned against the kitchen counter. "Okay."

Colleen heard the nervousness in his voice. "It's nothing bad, in fact I think you may be happy to hear what she told me."

Now she had Jeremy's full attention. She told him what Marcy had told her, about responsive versus spontaneous desire, and about how she was nervous that sex would still hurt, and that she felt so guilty about how she had avoided sex for so long, but also that she felt guilty about not getting help sooner. She told him she was willing to try what Marcy had suggested, to spend some time kissing and cuddling and see whether she experienced some arousal and the desire that hopefully would come with it. This all came out in a rush of words, and Jeremy listened, his face showing no reaction.

When she stopped talking, Jeremy didn't say a word. He just reached out and hugged her. They stood like that for what seemed like a long time.

"So now what?" Jeremy's voice was hopeful, but he didn't want to seem too eager to practice what Colleen had described.

"It's been a long day," Colleen said. For now, she was tired and just wanted to go to bed. "Can we try on the weekend?"

Jeremy was disappointed, but he didn't want to pressure her. "Okay, sure, whatever."

Touch is an essential part of overall well-being. Hand holding, hugging, kissing, and, yes, sex produce the "bonding" hormone oxytocin, which reduces stress hormones. There are also other "feel-good" hormones linked to oxytocin, so the importance of touch shouldn't be underestimated.

The weekend came and went, and despite Colleen's promise and Jeremy's hopefulness, they didn't spend much time together. And when they did, Colleen avoided getting within arm's length of Jeremy. He in turn avoided reminding her of the promise she'd made because he didn't want to start an argument. What he didn't know was that Colleen was thinking about this issue constantly, but her fear of experiencing pain was overwhelming. It was so bad that she called Marcy on Sunday night and left a message asking to push their appointment forward to Monday afternoon.

The nurse practitioner called her back early on Monday morning and arranged to see Colleen that afternoon, even though it was not a clinic day.

Colleen could not concentrate at work that morning. Thoughts whirled in her head as she prepared what she was going to tell Marcy. She looked at her watch often, willing the minutes and hours to pass but at the same time thinking of excuses to cancel the appointment. She knew none of this was rational, but she couldn't help herself.

She left her office early and showed up for the appointment an hour before she needed to. She sat in a coffee shop close to the cancer center, staring out the window as she thought about how she had messed up and let Marcy down. And Jeremy, of course—she had broken her promise to him, and she felt really bad about that.

She hadn't noticed that Marcy had entered the coffee shop, and now she was standing in front of her, a take-out cup in her hand.

"Hey, Colleen, are you waiting for our appointment?"

Colleen was startled and a little embarrassed to be caught unaware. "Yeah, I was."

"Do you want to start early? I popped in here to get some tea, but we can go back to my office if you're okay with that."

They chatted about the weather as they walked the short distance to the cancer center, but soon they were sitting in Marcy's office with the door closed.

"So, tell me why you wanted to change the day of this appointment. You sounded a little stressed on the voicemail you left."

Colleen took a deep breath and told the nurse what had happened since their last appointment just days before.

It was obvious to Marcy that Colleen was bothered by how she had avoided her husband and how guilty she felt about breaking her promise to him. "What do you think is holding you back, Colleen?"

"It's the pain! I just can't put myself through that again!" Colleen was on the verge of tears.

"Ah!" Marcy responded. "Of course you're scared of pain—anyone would be. But you're a long way from where you were months ago, and that time you tried to have sex may have been too soon. There is a real possibility that, with the right lubricant and by taking your time, sex or whatever you and Jeremy do is not going to hurt."

"Really?" Colleen's voice suggested she wasn't convinced.

"Okay, so remember that I'm not a sex therapist, but I have learned some things from other patients and from conferences I've attended over the years I've worked here." Marcy went on to explain to Colleen that, to help her understand that her body had healed, she needed to do some exploration of what kind of sexual touch felt good to her. She encouraged Colleen to spend some time alone and, using a good lubricant, to touch herself while doing some deep breathing and relaxation techniques that Marcy could show her. Alternatively, she could try this in the bath or the shower without lubricant. This could help Colleen experience how her body responded to genital touch.

"Do you think that will help?" Colleen seemed uncertain.

"It's worth a try, I would think," Marcy replied. "The status quo doesn't seem to be helping, right?"

"Yes, you're right," admitted Colleen. "Okay, I'll try."

People who try to have sex soon after treatment may find the experience is painful, and they might assume it will always be that way. Avoiding pain is a powerful motivation that leads to avoidance of all touch (see chapter 6). A positive first step is for cancer survivors to explore their body to find out what feels good, what doesn't, where there is pain or numbness, and to then guide their partner.

Once again, that evening Colleen repeated to Jeremy what Marcy had told her, but he didn't say much. He just nodded and went back to cutting vegetables for their dinner. Colleen was disappointed; she'd hoped he would be more interested in her progress, but she couldn't blame him for reacting less than enthusiastically. She waited until he was engrossed in a movie on TV then told him she was going to take a bath. She felt awkward about not telling him that she was going to follow Marcy's instructions, but she knew she had to do something to break the stalemate. The warm water of the bath was almost instantly relaxing, and she forgot for a minute why she was there. She started to touch herself, so gently at first that she barely felt anything, and then, as her confidence grew, with more pressure. It felt good, and there was no pain! To her surprise, she also felt something she hadn't felt in a long time. Was it possible she could be getting aroused? It seemed too good to be true after just one attempt, but there it was! She almost called out to Jeremy, but then she decided she wanted to keep this to herself for just a little bit longer. Telling him could wait till the weekend . . .

CONCLUSION

Loss of sexual desire is a common side effect of cancer treatment and is influenced by many factors, including pain with sexual activity, changes in body image, fear of recurrence, as well as depression and anxiety. Loss of desire may also occur in response to a decrease in sexual pleasure. If couples don't talk about these issues, there may be misunderstandings about the lack of sexual initiation—and this contributes to an overall lack of relationship satisfaction. Communicating about the situation may be enough to resolve any misunderstandings, but couples often need professional help both to start the conversation and to resolve their feelings.

TAKEAWAYS

- Sexual desire or libido is a cognitive experience that often changes over time or under specific circumstances. Physical changes, such as the loss of a breast or inability to have an erection, can affect body image and lower libido—or take it away completely.

- The intense desire that most people experience at the beginning of a relationship is called "limerence." It commonly fades over time as the novelty and excitement of a new partner decreases because life gets in the way!

- Couples often have different levels of desire; one person wants sex more or less often than the other, and this is a common reason for couples to seek professional help.

- Loss of desire may result in loss of everyday connection between the couple, including nonsexual displays of affection such as kissing and hugging.

- The partner of the cancer survivor may misinterpret the loss of desire as rejection or as due to something the partner has done, or as an indication the survivor is cheating.

- If these concerns aren't talked about, hurt feelings can lead to further misinterpretation, anger, and conflict. A professional such as a sex therapist may be needed to help the couple communicate their feelings and see the situation from the other's perspective.

- Communication is key to addressing issues—discuss your thoughts and questions with your partner, your doctor, your therapist, or a trusted family member or friend.

- There are lots of ways to address the absence of desire, and there are no reasons not to. A satisfying sex life can contribute to better overall well-being.

RECOMMENDED READING

For further reading, I recommend the following book:

Better Sex Through Mindfulness: How Women Can Cultivate Desire, by Lori A. Brotto

WEBSITES FOR ADDITIONAL INFORMATION

American Cancer Society
https://www.cancer.org/cancer/managing-cancer/side-effects/fertility-and-sexual-side-effects/sexuality-for-men-with-cancer/treatment-and-desire-and-response.html

CancerCare
https://www.cancercare.org/publications/292-intimacy_and_cancer

National Cancer Institute (NIH)
https://www.cancer.gov/about-cancer/treatment/side-effects/sexuality-men

CHAPTER 4

"Nothing's happening down there"

Problems with Arousal

Changes in arousal are common and cause distress to individuals and their partners. In men, changes in or loss of erections impacts not only sexual performance but also masculine self-image and sense of masculinity. Up to 95% of men treated for prostate cancer report erectile problems.[1] Among women with gynecologic cancer treated with radiation therapy, 40% to 90% report decreased arousal.[2] If vaginal lubrication is not adequate or is missing, penetration is painful to the point where it may be impossible. For both men and women, arousal is a product of hormones, nerves, and blood vessels responding in concert; not surprisingly, damage to these from cancer treatment creates challenges that may negatively impact sexual relationships.

PAUL AND TINA

Paul and Tina have faced their share of challenges over almost 40 years of marriage. They struggled to have children before adopting their twin boys, who are now in their 30s with children of their own. In 1987, the couple lost their entire savings in the stock market crash, and Tina had to go back to work as a nurse.

Tina lost both her parents in a car crash when she and Paul were newly married, and as an only child, she hasn't had any family support over the years. Now in their mid-60s, Paul and Tina had reached a stage in their lives when their primary focus could be travel and spending time with their grandchildren.

But their challenges continued when Paul was diagnosed with intermediate-risk prostate cancer. The diagnosis was not unexpected; his primary care provider had discussed the probability of this when they'd talked about the results of the MRI and prostate biopsy he'd had after his annual PSA had risen rapidly. The urologist who'd done the biopsy was one of the best in the city according to Paul's primary care provider, Dr. Jameson. The urologist had also performed the robotic radical prostatectomy that Paul had been offered. The doctor had reassured Paul that the surgery had been successful and that "he had spared the nerves on both sides." The nerves involved in erections run on the outside of the prostate gland, and not destroying these nerves during surgery is thought to preserve erectile function.

Paul didn't experience any problems during the weeks of recovery from surgery. He had always exercised at least three times a week and prided himself on being the same weight as when he'd gotten married. He credited his fitness for his and Tina's continued sexual relationship, which hadn't changed much, if at all, over the years of their marriage. Until now . . .

Their 40th anniversary was six weeks after his surgery and, as usual, he wanted to celebrate the milestone with a special dinner and sex afterward. Tina was concerned; she had heard from one of her friends whose husband had had the same surgery that "things in that department" had changed. Her friend hadn't said anything more, but that was enough for Tina to worry. She wasn't concerned for herself since, after menopause, her desire was not what it used to be, but she was worried this was going to be a big deal for Paul.

Things did not go well the night of their anniversary. Dinner was fine, but that was the only success of the night. Paul wasn't able to have an erection, no matter what they tried, and he left the bedroom to spend the night on the couch. Tina pleaded with him to come back to bed, but he lay with his eyes closed, his head on the armrest of the couch, and didn't even respond to her. The next morning, he refused to talk about it and went to the gym without his usual coffee. He seemed to be in a better mood when he came back from the gym.

Tina tried to talk to him again. "Honey, it's really soon, just six weeks from your surgery . . . Let's wait a while, and I'm sure it'll get better."

Paul just grunted.

She tried again. "I hope you're not upset because of me."

"I'm upset because of *me*! The surgeon said that he spared the nerves and that everything was going to be fine."

Paul rarely raised his voice, and Tina was taken aback at his outburst. It was better than his silence but surprising nonetheless.

Up to 95% of men will not be able to achieve erections six months after surgery for prostate cancer, despite their pre-surgery erectile function. Results for men treated with radiation alone are slightly better at 88%.[1] The most important predictor is the man's erectile function *before* treatment; if he had problems with erections before treatment, chances of recovery of erections are very small. But good erections presurgery is not a guarantee that function will be anywhere as good after surgery.

Tina offered to attend Paul's follow-up visit with the urologist the next week. Paul didn't reply, and Tina read his silence as rejection. She understood he was upset, but the night before was the first and only time that something like this had happened. She was convinced it was too early for him to have recovered sexual function, but he needed to find this out for himself.

Many men have unrealistic expectations of sexual recovery after prostate cancer surgery. It's important that they receive accurate information before the surgery and information about treatment options, but that doesn't mean they shouldn't have hope or a belief that their recovery will be different from the norm! Including the survivor's sexual partner in this discussion is very important.

Paul came back from the appointment with his urologist looking dejected.

"Don't even ask!" he almost barked at Tina. "He said that it'll take time, and I should be happy that the pathology looks good and he got all the cancer."

That was Tina's major concern—that the cancer had been removed entirely—but she knew she shouldn't say much, if anything, about it. Paul's focus seemed to be on his erections alone.

But the situation did not improve. They tried to have sex twice more in the next month, and each time he grew frustrated and then angry at the lack of change. It was now three months after the surgery, and despite Tina's promises that this wasn't affecting her, Paul wasn't convinced. And he didn't want to talk about it, no matter what she said.

It's important that the man and his sexual partner talk about the potential for sexual problems after surgery, as well as the possible emotional impacts of these changes. If the partners don't talk openly about this, misunderstandings and resentment may build up, as they had started to for this couple. Open communication can often head off more difficult conversations down the line, and when partners share the burden, often there can be more understanding—and less stress.

The silence between Paul and Tina continued. This was distressing for Tina; they had always been able to talk about anything and everything. Soon it was time for Paul's six-month appointment, and once again, he refused to have Tina go with him. He came back from this appointment even angrier than before.

"I didn't even see the guy who did the surgery! I saw this young person, his PA or something, and he also told me it was too early! When is it going to be too late?"

Just 43% of men, even those in their 50s and early 60s, see a return of erections the same as they had before their prostate surgery,[3] and their sexual satisfaction remains low despite this. Treatment for erectile dysfunction is available; a stepwise approach is suggested, with oral medications (Viagra, Cialis, Levitra, or Stendra) as initial treatment.[4] Other treatments include the penile pump,[5] penile injections,[6] or penile implant.[7]

"Did you ask to see the urologist?" Tina asked. "The PA, the physician assistant, works under the physician's direction." Tina couldn't stop herself from trying to calm him, even though, as her words came out, she knew this was not going to help. She tried again. "Maybe Dr. Jameson can help . . ." Dr. Jameson was their primary care provider, and they both trusted and liked him very much.

"Hmm," Paul responded. It was not easy for him to ask for help, and talking about sexual problems was especially difficult, but he knew he couldn't continue with the status quo.

He made an appointment to see Dr. Jameson later that week. He came home from the appointment looking more hopeful. His doctor had given him a prescription for Viagra, and he felt optimistic it could work. Tina was secretly worried, however, as a friend's husband had tried the same thing with poor results.

"He gave me a prescription for 'the little blue pill,' and I left it at the drugstore," Paul said. "It'll be ready later this afternoon. I really hope it works."

"Me too, honey," Tina replied, but she wasn't sure. Her friend, the one with the husband who'd had the same surgery, had told her that nothing had helped, and the little blue pill had just given him a bad headache. Plus, he'd started taking the pills right after his surgery, unlike Paul.

To Paul's disappointment, the medication did not help. Tina tried to keep his hope alive by looking on the internet for alternative treatments. What she found was not appealing—most other treatments were more invasive and didn't show great success. When she shared the information with Paul, he shuddered. Tina didn't say so, but she was disappointed as well—this was clearly affecting her too.

"There is no way I'm going to use a pump or an injection into my penis!" Paul said. "I just have to accept that part of my life is over."

It's my life too, Tina thought but didn't say out loud.

Nothing changed over the next several months. It was now 18 months since Paul's surgery, and he had one more follow-up appointment with the urologist, his last one. His future care would be with his primary care provider. According to Paul, the urologist seemed defensive when Paul told him that, firstly, his erections had not returned, and secondly, he had tried the pill prescribed by Dr. Jameson, but that too hadn't helped. The urologist didn't offer any other advice—he just wished Paul well and then left the exam room.

"I wonder if Dr. Jameson may have some other suggestions . . ." Tina saw how despondent Paul was, and she wasn't sure they could continue with their present situation. His self-image appeared to be suffering in all aspects, and she couldn't ignore this. He seemed to have lost interest in most activities, even in spending time with their beloved grandchildren. She insisted on going with him to see Dr. Jameson; there was a chance that Paul wouldn't tell Dr. Jameson how he was really feeling, and Tina might need to speak up . . .

Men may experience depression because of their loss of sexual function (see chapter 7), as well as changes to their masculine self-image and self-esteem, and even feelings of shame. In Paul's case, seeking out a mental health-care provider would at least help with his mood. Assembling a team of practitioners isn't just essential for cancer treatment while it's happening; a good team is also important when dealing with the consequences of cancer treatment. Sex therapists are readily available in many locations, but the key is to start somewhere and to find practitioners willing to help.

Paul reluctantly agreed to the plan for Tina to go with him to see Dr. Jameson. In the days before the appointment, she wrote down a list of questions in case, in the moment, she forgot what she wanted to ask. She hoped Dr. Jameson would have the time to answer what was now quite a long list.

"Nice to see you, Tina!" the doctor said, welcoming them into his office. "And Paul? How are things with you?" He was careful to not ask specifically about the medication he had prescribed Paul; he hoped Tina knew about it, but perhaps Paul hadn't told her or hadn't taken any pills.

"It's okay, Doc, Tina knows. I'm only here because she insisted that I see you and that she come with me."

"Good. This affects her too, as you know." Dr Jameson gave a small smile. "You know what they say—happy wife, happy life. But neither of you look very happy. So, tell me why you're here today."

Paul looked at Tina and nodded, encouraging her to share her thoughts.

"The pills haven't worked, Dr. Jameson, and I read how you're—I mean, the man is—supposed to take them an hour before sexual activity. And also that, um, stimulation is needed. We did all that but still nothing."

The doctor asked Paul whether he was interested in other interventions and mentioned a urologist with a special interest in sexual medicine who could offer injections or a penile implant.

"Absolutely not!" Paul's voice was loud, and Tina was startled at how vehement he was. "I am not interested in any of that stuff! They all sound, well, painful . . . Are there no herbs or something like that I can try?"

Before the physician could answer, Tina spoke. "I read about something called 'shock therapy' or stem cells."

"Funny you should mention that," Dr. Jameson said. "I was just reading an article in a journal about new treatments for erection issues, and it said that it's too early to consider shock-wave therapy or using stem cells. There just isn't enough evidence to support their use, especially in men like Paul who have been treated for prostate cancer. And herbal supplements aren't useful either. It's disappointing, I know, but I have something to suggest."

Paul and Tina were looking at him intently.

"Another article in the same medical journal showed that for some men and their partner something called 'mindfulness meditation' can be helpful. It's noninvasive, of course, and has also been shown to help with anxiety and negative thinking. Is this something you would consider?"

"I certainly would!" Tina was quick to respond. "But it's up to Paul . . ."

Paul wasn't sure, but he also realized it might help and wouldn't hurt. "I guess we can give it a try. How do we go about it?"

Mindfulness meditation (see appendix 1) has been shown to improve sexual satisfaction and help men move away from a focus on sexual performance.

"I can give you a copy of the article," said Dr. Jameson, "but I also know a therapist who uses mindfulness approaches to sexual difficulties. Would you be interested in a referral to her?"

Paul was still skeptical—what good would a therapist do when medication hadn't helped? But Tina was nodding her head in agreement.

Paul shrugged. Sure, he could give it a try.

JANET AND BRUCE

Janet, who is 52 years old, lives with her partner Bruce, aged 58. Neither of them wanted to get married again, having experienced painful divorces in the past. Two years ago, they met on a cruise, where Janet was celebrating her divorce and Bruce was traveling with his elderly mother, who'd wanted to see Vietnam but hadn't been well enough to travel alone. The attraction between Janet and Bruce had been immediate. Within months of arriving home, Janet had moved 500 miles to the city where Bruce lived. She worked in IT, so she had no problem relocating and continuing her job remotely. It was hard leaving her friends but, in her eyes, love was more important, especially after her troubled marriage.

Soon after moving in with Bruce, she started experiencing rectal bleeding every now and then. She hadn't yet found a doctor and mostly ignored the bleeding, assuming she had hemorrhoids. A year went by, and she finally recognized she needed to do something about the bleeding. She went to an urgent care clinic, and they ordered a colonoscopy; within three weeks she found herself in an oncologist's office. The colonoscopy showed a tumor in her large intestine, and she needed treatment with chemotherapy and eventually surgery to remove the tumor and adjacent bowel.

She had a rough time with the treatments, spending most days in bed and rising only to go to appointments. Through it all, Bruce cared for her with compassion and patience. Their relationship was still relatively new, but he proved to her that he was there for the long haul, and she was grateful and determined to repay him once she was well again.

Recovery from the surgery took longer than she expected, but she was relieved she didn't need to have an ostomy. Her energy level was low, which frustrated her because she was eager to get back to exercising. And then there was the issue of sex— or rather the lack of it. Before her diagnosis, they'd had an active sex life, something they both treasured because, in their previous relationships, sex had been problematic. When they'd gotten together, neither had anticipated how wonderful sex could be, so the absence of this experience during and after her treatment was a loss for both of them. Bruce didn't complain or even mention it, but Janet could sense how it bothered him, and it bothered her too!

One Saturday morning, Janet decided they needed to at least try to make love. She'd been told by one of the nurses that they needed to be "careful" about sex while she was having chemotherapy. When she'd asked what "careful" meant, the nurse had told her they needed to use condoms for intercourse, but she hadn't said for how long or even why. This had confused Janet at the time, but she hadn't been feeling up for sex, so it had been a moot point. But now Janet was no longer having chemotherapy, and it was time they did something.

Most people having chemotherapy are advised to avoid penetrative intercourse or use a barrier (condom or dental dam) for 36 to 48 hours after each treatment for a number of reasons. One of them is to avoid the partner being exposed to the breakdown products of the chemotherapy that may be present in body fluids. Another reason is that chemotherapy often weakens the immune system; intercourse and oral sex may pose an infection risk to the person with cancer.

Disappointment followed. What used to be mutually satisfying for Janet and Bruce was anything but. In fact, what happened was worse than either of them could have imagined. When Bruce tried to enter her vagina, Janet pushed him off, her facial expression showing how much it hurt. Her whole body contracted into a fetal position, and tears streamed down her cheeks. Bruce immediately put his arms around her and hugged her without saying anything. He waited for her to explain what she was feeling. After a few minutes, he felt her relax, and she turned to him.

"What happened?" Bruce asked softly. "Was it pain or something else?"

For a few seconds Janet struggled to describe what she was feeling, but then she found the words. "It was like I was being stabbed with a shard of glass! I am so sorry, this wasn't your fault . . . I thought I was ready, but obviously I'm not."

"Shhhh, love . . . we'll figure this out." Bruce's mind whirled. He didn't understand, but he could see how upset she was, and he was determined to help her find help.

When they were dressed, they sat at the kitchen table, mugs of hot tea in front of them, and talked.

"I guess I need to talk to someone about this, but who?" Janet wasn't sure who might be able to explain and, more importantly, help her.

"Maybe your surgeon?" Bruce wasn't sure either.

"I'm seeing him next week . . ."

The appointment with the surgeon was quick, as usual. He was running late—an emergency, his receptionist explained—and Janet didn't want to delay him further. As he was about to leave the exam room, she took a deep breath and asked him why sex was so painful.

He seemed shocked at the question, and his reply was curt. "You'll have to ask your oncologist. The surgery could not be the cause—entirely different part of your anatomy."

The resident, a young woman who was working with him, waited for him to leave the room before she spoke. "Janet, may I call you by your first name? Okay, so you really should speak to your oncologist. But here's a question—are you postmenopausal? I know this is a weird question coming from a surgical resident, but it may be important."

Janet had to think for a moment. In the months of her recovery, she hadn't really noticed, but on thinking about it, she realized she hadn't had a period for ages. She vaguely remembered that someone, her oncologist maybe, had told her the chemotherapy would push her into menopause. She understood that to mean she wouldn't have periods anymore, but that was all she recalled. She hadn't thought about that detail since . . . how long had it been?

"I guess I am postmenopausal," Janet said. "I haven't had a period since my chemo . . ."

"Chemo often causes a whole lot of side effects," the resident continued, "including menopause for many women, especially those who are close to the age of normal menopause. I know this because I did some time in the gynecology clinic last year. The loss of estrogen may be what caused the pain you had. There's a special clinic that deals with these issues, and you don't need a referral to go there. Are you interested?"

"Yes, please!"

Chemotherapy is designed to attack cancer cells, which divide rapidly. There are many other cells in our body that divide rapidly, including those in the ovaries, where the majority of estrogen is produced. Chemotherapy causes the onset of menopause by shutting down the ovaries, and this can be temporary or permanent. The closer a woman is to the usual age of menopause—the early 50s for most women—the more likely the ovaries will stop producing estrogen. Loss of estrogen contributes to the thinning of the vaginal walls and to a decrease in natural bodily lubrication, necessary for comfortable sexual

intercourse. In many cases, finding the right lubricant can ease
the pain of intercourse and make it enjoyable again.

Janet called the clinic as soon as she got home. She booked
an appointment for the following Wednesday evening—a sched-
uling bonus for working women, she thought.

Wednesday came quickly, and she found the clinic in a new
building on the medical-school campus. From the outside the
clinic looked quite austere, but inside it was nicely decorated
with desert-sand-colored furnishings and walls. She was ush-
ered into an office, not an examination room, by a friendly
woman who said she was a volunteer. Within minutes a woman
about her own age entered the room.

"Hi, hello! I'm Nancy, one of the NPs—nurse practitioners—
here. How are you today?"

"Um, okay, I guess."

"Well, let's see if I can move the needle to more than okay!"

Nancy smiled as she spoke, and Janet relaxed a little. She'd
been thinking a lot about her care over the previous months,
and while most of the medical team treating her had been efficient, there hadn't been much warmth from most of them. And
there was a lot she hadn't been told, she now realized.

"So, please tell me—what brings you to us this evening?"

Janet wasn't sure where to start, but she decided to open with
a question. "Is it normal for someone like me to go into menopause because of cancer?" The question hadn't come out exactly
as she'd intended, but she was nervous.

"So, you've had cancer?" the nurse practitioner asked. "Can
you tell me what kind and what treatment you had?"

Janet answered her but didn't not stop there. She found herself describing what had happened over the course of the previous months. The nurse practitioner listened closely; she didn't

make notes or look at anything other than Janet's face. She nodded every now and then, a sympathetic look on her face.

"Okay, what you describe, the pain with penetration, or
rather with an attempt at penetration, sounds typical for a dry
and very sore vagina and vulva. I have some practical suggestions for you to start with, and then we can move to other issues if you want."

"Yes, please and thank you!" Janet felt her pulse beating fast.
Here was some help!

*Reduced levels of estrogen in the blood result in loss of lubrication,
and this causes pain with sexual touch of the vulva as well as pain
with vaginal penetration. The body responds to pain by tightening
the muscles of the pelvic floor (see chapter 6).*

Nancy stood up and reached onto a shelf behind Janet. She
pulled down a basket that contained a collection of tubes and
bottles as well as some pamphlets.

"This here is my basket of tricks! Well, nothing here is really
a trick. There are a lot of products available to help women
manage the discomfort—no, correct that—the *pain* that they
experience as a result of the dryness due to the loss of estrogen. Menopause is a normal stage of life for women—it's not a
disease—but for women who have a chemically induced menopause because of chemotherapy, the symptoms can be worse."

For the next 15 minutes, Janet watched and listened as Nancy
gave her what she called her "menopause show-and-tell."

*Moisturizers can be useful products to help with external (vulvar)
and internal (vaginal) dryness. Lubricants are vital for comfort when
vaginal penetration is the goal. Most of those available at a drugstore*

and without a prescription are hormone-free. Take care to use only products that do not contain irritants. If these products don't alleviate the pain, you can consider prescription medications. Chapter 12 offers details on both nonhormonal and prescription-required medications.

"I have some samples of moisturizers and lubricants if you'd like to take some home," Nancy continued. "I'd like to see you again in a couple of weeks when you've had time to try some or all of them, and we can then decide where to go next if needed. How does that sound?"

"That sounds great, more than great really! Can I bring my partner next time? I'm not sure that I'll remember everything you told me, and he needs to hear what I hear, right?"

"You're 100% right on that. Sure, you can bring him—I'd like to meet this man you've talked about. He sounds special."

Janet got up from the chair, the samples Nancy had offered in her hand. There was a definite lightness in her step as she left the room. She couldn't wait to tell Bruce about the appointment. And to try out the samples!

CONCLUSION

Problems with arousal for both men and women are common after cancer treatment. The cause may be alterations to nerves, resulting in erectile dysfunction in men, or destruction of blood vessels, resulting in loss of lubrication in women. While treatments are available, they don't always work and may have side effects. In addition, some people may assume these effects are to be expected after treatment, and so they don't seek help. As with other sexual problems, the partner's involvement is key to managing or solving the issue—and so is asking for help from a health-care provider.

TAKEAWAYS

- Sexual arousal in men is visible in the form of an erection. In women, arousal isn't visible because it's experienced as vaginal lubrication, which is internal.

- Women can have penetration in the absence of physical arousal, but men cannot have intercourse without an erection.

- Loss of erections often affects the man's masculine self-image and may impact the couple's relationship.

- The cause of the loss of erections is physical after treatment for prostate cancer, and possibly after treatment for other cancers involving the pelvis, but emotional distress often occurs as well and further complicates the situation.

- Vaginal lubrication is a sign of arousal in women and is produced by estrogen in the bloodstream. Loss of estrogen in the vaginal tissues results in a decrease in lubrication and pain with sexual touch or penetration.

- Pain with sexual touch or penetration results in loss of sexual interest for many women.

WEBSITES FOR ADDITIONAL INFORMATION

American Cancer Society

https://www.cancer.org/cancer/managing-cancer/side
-effects/fertility-and-sexual-side-effects/sexuality-for
-men-with-cancer/erections-and-treatment.html

Breastcancer.org

https://www.breastcancer.org/treatment-side-effects
/vaginal-dryness/moisturizers-lubricants

Johns Hopkins Medicine

https://www.hopkinsmedicine.org/health/wellness
-and-prevention/life-after-cancer-changes-to-a-mans
-sex-life

National Cancer Institute (NIH)

https://www.cancer.gov/about-cancer/treatment/side
-effects/sexuality-men

OncoLink

https://www.oncolink.org/support/sexuality-fertility
/sexuality/erectile-dysfunction-after-cancer-treatment
https://www.oncolink.org/support/sexuality-fertility
/sexuality/vaginal-dryness-and-painful-intercourse

Prostate Cancer Foundation

https://www.pcf.org/about-prostate-cancer/prostate
-cancer-side-effects/erectile-dysfunction/

CHAPTER 5

"What's the point if I feel nothing?"

Changes in Orgasms

Many cancer survivors find that sexual activity feels different since their treatment, and they may experience altered sensations, including difficulty reaching orgasm. Half of the women with breast cancer in a study reported changes in their ability to have or quality of orgasms.[1,2] Those who regularly experienced orgasms before cancer, either through masturbation or intercourse, may find their orgasms are now elusive or absent. This affects not just the survivor but their sexual partner too.

CHRIS AND BETHANY

Chris, a 24-year-old graduate student, had been diagnosed with acute myeloid leukemia and had a stem cell transplant a year ago. One of his nurses, Bethany, became his girlfriend; they'd been dating for three months, since meeting up again after his discharge from hospital. He was doing well and had plans to return to university for the fall semester. Bethany had been a great support, and he was grateful he didn't have to explain anything to her related to his illness or transplant—she understood what he'd gone through. With her encouragement, he started to attend a monthly support group of young-adult survivors. He'd been reluctant at first, but now he found it really helpful to hear how other young adults like him were coping after treatment. He became good friends with a guy his age, Jared, who'd had his transplant a couple of months before Chris. They had a lot in common, but Jared was more extroverted and outspoken at support-group meetings.

At the last support-group meeting, Jared talked about his dating struggles. He described his loss of confidence after failing to maintain an erection on two separate occasions with two different women he'd met online. Chris was a little shocked that Jared could talk about this so openly, but he also thought it was brave, and the others attending the meeting responded with words of encouragement. What Chris did not contribute to the discussion was that he too was experiencing a problem—he wasn't ready to talk about it. Not even to Bethany . . .

It's not easy for most people to talk openly about sexual or relationship concerns. Support groups, where others who have experienced the same diagnosis and often the same treatments, can be a safe space to share even the most private concerns. But not everyone is ready to share with others, and an experienced facilitator is key to maintaining the safety of all participants.

During the coffee break at the meeting, Jared approached Chris. "Hey, buddy, you seemed surprised when I told the group I was having some problems. Why was that?"

Jared's question surprised Chris. He hadn't been aware Jared had picked up on his reaction. "Um, I just didn't expect anyone to be that open about, well, sex stuff. I mean, it's really brave and all that, and the group was super supportive . . ." Chris wasn't sure what he was supposed to say to his new friend. It was great he could talk openly about something so private, but it wasn't something Chris saw himself as ever being able to do.

"Hey, if it can happen to me, it can happen to any guy!" Jared wasn't letting go of the topic despite Chris's growing discomfort.

"I guess so," Chris responded, ending the conversation.

At his next appointment with the transplant team, Chris saw the social worker, Nancy. He hadn't spoken to her since his discharge, and she greeted him with her usual warmth, which hid a directness that was key to her role.

"Hi, Chris! So good to see you—it feels like it's been ages. And look at that!" She looked down at the iPad she was carrying, checking the details of the clinic appointments for the day. "It's been a year since your transplant! How are you doing? A little bird told me that you and one of the nurses from the unit are hanging out a little more than is medically indicated!" She had a broad grin on her face as she said the last part, but she was keyed in to the transplant-unit gossip, so of course she knew about him and Bethany.

"Yeah, Bethany and I connected a couple of months ago." Chris blushed as he admitted this.

"How's it going?" Nancy asked. She was genuinely interested, having seen some nurse-patient relationships in the past that had not gone well.

"It's fairly new and, so far, it's really good. She understands what I've gone through, you know? We're taking it slow, but I really like her and she likes me . . . or at least it seems she does!"

"I'm really happy for you, Chris, and for Bethany too. She's lovely, and I hope things go well for you."

Chris didn't know what more to say. Nancy had opened the door for him to talk about his relationship, but he was hesitant. Should he tell her what was going on, or rather what was *not* happening? She had been helpful after his transplant while he'd still been in hospital and had been despondent about having to take time off from his studies. But she was a woman, and he was having a sexual problem that he didn't understand . . .

While it may seem obvious that if you have a sexual problem you should talk to someone of the same sex, this isn't always true. An empathetic and knowledgeable professional of the opposite sex won't make assumptions based on their own experiences. They may prove to be useful in asking clarifying questions that help to identify all aspects of the problem and help you to find a potential solution. And medical professionals in particular are educated in how the whole body works, so even if they don't have deep knowledge or expertise in the area, they can often point you to someone who does.

Chris knew he needed help before he and Bethany started a sexual relationship, so he took a deep breath and told Nancy what was happening. He told her that he knew it would take time to recover from his illness, but he hadn't expected to experience sexual changes after his transplant. He told her that, while he wasn't sexually active at this time, he hadn't had an orgasm with masturbation, and he was concerned this was going to be a problem for the rest of his life.

Nancy listened as he talked, her face reflecting the seriousness of what he was disclosing. "Of course you're worried, Chris, and thank you for sharing this. You know that anything you tell me is in the strictest confidence. I'm not a sex therapist or sexual-medicine specialist, but I have heard similar stories from other survivors. Would it be okay if I referred you to someone who can help?"

"I guess so, but can this be fixed? What's wrong with me?"

Chris's voice was shaky, and while he was relieved to hear Nancy had heard of something similar, he still felt as though he were the only person this was happening to.

"There's a sex therapist that I've referred other patients to . . . I can call her today and see if she's taking on new clients."

Nancy was making a note on her iPad, and even though he wanted to tell her to not bother with the referral, part of him felt that getting help was the best thing he could do. He really liked Bethany, and he had a feeling she was ready to take their relationship further—and that meant sex was the next step. He was pretty sure she would notice if he didn't have an orgasm . . . and of course he was really worried there was something seriously wrong with him. What was happening was weird, he thought, because in all other ways he was "normal." He was attracted to Bethany, and he was having erections when they fooled around, and at other times too, so why was an orgasm so elusive?

By the time he got home after seeing his oncologist, there was an email from Nancy with the name and contact information for the sex therapist she had talked about. The therapist, Dr. Golden, would be happy to see him, according to Nancy. Before he lost his nerve, Chris called her office and made an appointment for the following week. He was glad he didn't have to wait long as he was sure he'd be tempted to cancel the appointment if it were weeks away.

He didn't tell Bethany any of this, and she didn't ask about his appointments as a rule. She'd told him that she wanted to be his girlfriend and not a nurse in their relationship, and this had sounded like a good idea to him too.

The day of the appointment arrived. Dr. Golden appeared to be in her 50s. She was of average height and wore a brightly colored dress. Her dark hair fell to her shoulders, and a pair of tortoiseshell glasses on top of her head kept her bangs off her face. Her office was filled with sunlight from large windows overlooking a small garden. Bookshelves covered the remaining three walls, and there were piles of books on the floor.

Chris couldn't help smiling as he sat on a worn leather couch and looked around; he imagined that one day he might have an office just like this.

Dr. Golden didn't apologize for what some would call a mess, and instead she got right to the point. "Nancy told me a little bit about your history . . . stem cell transplant for acute myeloid leukemia, about a year ago, right? You're a graduate student in something to do with the environment, and you're having a problem."

Chris couldn't help blinking as she frankly recited his history. What else had Nancy told her? "Uh, yes, that's correct."

"So how can I help you? Or at least try to help you." Dr. Golden leaned forward, closing the space between them, but it wasn't threatening in any way. Rather, she seemed intently interested in what he was going to say next.

Chris hesitated for a few seconds, not sure where to start.

"Listen, you need to speak plainly if we're to get anywhere." Dr. Golden wasn't wasting any time. "Please don't try to beat around the bush. There is nothing to be embarrassed about. I've pretty much heard all the words when it comes to sex, so go ahead—what's going on, or not?"

"Okay, so I haven't been able to have an . . . you know, an orgasm, since my transplant."

There, it was out in the open. It was the second time he'd said the words, both times to women who were as old as his mother, and he had survived!

"Ah. Nancy didn't tell me that, just that you could do with seeing me. So can I ask you some additional questions?"

Chris nodded. He felt more comfortable responding to questions rather than describing outright what he was experiencing.

The therapist asked him whether this was happening when he masturbated (yes) and when he was with a partner (not yet); she also asked about when this had started (it had been happening ever since his transplant). Then she asked whether he was he using pornography when he masturbated (blushing, he replied that yes, he was).

Dr. Golden appeared to be thinking about something, and she was silent for a moment. "Have you noticed any changes in sensation of your hands or fingers?"

This seemed a strange question to Chris, but he realized that yes, he had been having some problems using the keyboard of his computer, but he'd thought that was because he wasn't typing all the time since he'd put his university courses on hold. "My fingertips are a bit numb. They told me this might happen after all the chemotherapy."

Certain chemotherapy agents cause nerve damage, usually to hands and feet, but the damage may also affect the genitals. This damage may cause numbness or tingling, and in medical terms it's called "peripheral neuropathy."

Dr. Golden explained these side effects to Chris. "It's possible that you have some nerve damage to the skin of your genitals, resulting in loss of sensation," she continued. "My understanding is that this is a side effect of some kinds of chemotherapy, but I don't know exactly what treatments you had."

Chris was puzzled. Why had no one told him about this? Or maybe they had, and he hadn't paid attention in the shock of the diagnosis and admission to hospital for the transplant.

Dr. Golden interrupted his thoughts. "But let's talk about what you can do about this. That seems rather more important to me than the cause—we can't change what happened in the past, can we?"

Chris nodded and focused on what she said next.

"There is always more than one factor when it comes to sex. When you've not been able to have an orgasm, it often becomes a cycle, so the next time you masturbate, or have intercourse, you set yourself up for not having an orgasm. In sex therapy, it's called 'performance anxiety,' even though sex should not be considered a performance! Does that make sense?"

Chris nodded again. But he was still anxious about this and the possibility that the problem wasn't going to go away.

"You may find that when you and your girlfriend start a sexual relationship, things will be different. There is novelty with a new partner, and being with someone you care about makes for a more erotic experience compared to masturbation. But the key is to control your mind and the anxiety around whether you will have an orgasm or not."

Chris hadn't considered this before. He'd been thinking that he had a purely mechanical problem, that he was not doing something the right way.

The therapist continued. "When you're anxious, you're not fully present in the moment—and also not focused on sensation. If you aren't fully aware of the sensations, the message doesn't go to your brain that you're experiencing pleasure, and then the brain doesn't trigger the physical sensation of orgasm."

"So, it's kind of a loop?"

"Yes. Exactly. Now we need to talk about being focused on sensation by being fully in the moment and shutting off negative thoughts."

"Is there some way to test my skin's sensitivity?" Chris's analytical mind was looking for proof of the nerve damage.

"I don't think you need any testing at the moment, but if what I suggest you try doesn't work, we can look at more medical strategies. How does that sound?"

Chris nodded in agreement. The idea of someone "testing" his genitals did not sound like something he'd enjoy!

"I am going to give you some suggestions for relaxation and being in the moment, both when masturbating and when you're with your partner," Dr. Golden said. "You may also want to consider using a vibrator externally on the penis or scrotum to increase the intensity of sensations, overcoming any negative thoughts you may be experiencing."

"Guys can use a vibrator?" Chris had never heard of this before; he knew that women used them, but men? This was something interesting . . .

Using a vibrator (see chapter 12) on the penis, scrotum, or perineum (the area between the scrotum and anus) can elicit intensely pleasurable sensations that override so-called performance anxiety. Many men are not aware of this, but it can be a simple solution to a complex mind-body problem. Vibrators are available through online stores such as Amazon, as well as in many major retailers and sex stores.

Dr. Golden had another question. "Are you using a lubricant or lotion when you masturbate?"

"Yes, I use hand lotion—or soap if I'm in the shower." He blushed as he replied; he'd never talked so openly about anything like this.

"It may be that you need more friction, and lotion, soap, or lube decrease friction. This may seem contradictory, because for penis-in-vagina intercourse, lube makes intercourse better for many women. And less friction delays orgasm for the man, which many couples find is a good thing. But we can talk more about that in the future, when you're sexually active with your partner."

Chris looked at his watch. The appointment was almost over, and he wanted to go home and see if Dr. Golden's suggestions worked. It was time to experiment, and then do some online shopping for a vibrator!

SOFIA AND BAILEY

Her family and friends had been shocked when Sofia was diagnosed with breast cancer at just 27 years of age, but no one had been more shocked than Sofia herself. She'd never heard of any women her age with this cancer, and even the name of the cancer clinic she attended—the Morningstar Young Adult Cancer Clinic—emphasized that she was still a young adult. But cancer was only supposed to happen to older people! Her partner, Bailey, reminded her when she was in the midst of treatment that cancer didn't discriminate, but that didn't help Sofia feel any better.

She and Bailey argued a lot during treatment, stupid fights about little things that shouldn't have resulted in shouting followed by wounded silence. Sofia admitted she was fortunate to not need chemotherapy, and she got through the radiation following the lumpectomy with what seemed like just a slight sunburn on the side of her chest. But she was still angry this had happened to her at a time when everything had been going well—she had just started a great new job, and her relationship with Bailey had been so good that they'd started looking to buy a house together. Then boom! Cancer and surgery and radiation and the realization that bad things happen to good people.

When cancer affects someone between the ages of 19 and 35 (or 39 in some places), it's considered to be young-adult cancer. Because of the significant milestones people typically reach during this stage of life—establishing a career and starting and maintaining sexual relationships, among others—cancer during these years can cause major disruptions and challenges.

Sofia had never been an angry person before her diagnosis. She had a public-facing career as a curator for a small art gallery; one of the reasons she chose this role was that she loved interacting with clients who were interested in the visual arts. Now every day was a struggle as she had to pretend to be outgoing and bubbly, but what she really wanted to do was smash something. Hiding how she felt was exhausting, and when she came home after work, all she wanted to do was crawl into bed and watch movies on her iPad.

Bailey was growing increasingly frustrated with her behavior. Their relationship was almost a year old, and this was not what Bailey had imagined life with Sofia would be like. She'd fallen in love with Sofia because of her sunny nature, and this 180-degree change wasn't something she'd ever thought would happen.

She tried to figure out how she could help Sofia, first by asking at regular intervals how her partner was feeling and whether she was depressed. This was not helpful and ended up in another one of their fights.

Bailey tried another tactic. "What are you most worried about? Maybe talking about it will help . . ."

Yet another fight ensued, and this time it ended with Sofia slamming their bedroom door shut and Bailey sleeping on the couch.

Bailey had bought a couple of self-help books online that claimed to offer insight into cancer survivorship for women with breast cancer. But they remained stacked and unread on a shelf in the hall closet. She thought about talking to Sofia's mother or sister, but their relationship with Sofia also seemed to be going through a rough patch. Bailey was at her wit's end, and she wasn't sure how long she'd be able to endure things the way they were.

While acute depression is not unusual at the time of diagnosis (see chapter 7) and is regarded as a reaction to a life-threatening situation, not everyone experiences depression. Anxiety is also common and can persist for months or even years, as fears of a cancer recurrence persist (see chapter 7). People's responses to a diagnosis vary; some people will be angry, and others will use the experience as an opportunity for personal growth or a greater appreciation of life.

One afternoon, Sofia came home in tears—she'd been called out by the owner of the art gallery for being rude to one of their best clients. Sofia had talked about this particular client in the past, and not in a complimentary way; he was, in her words, "entitled and self-important." The client had complained to Sofia's boss about the way she'd spoken to him. Her boss had then reprimanded her and suggested she take the rest of the day off.

Bailey saw this as an opportunity to suggest to Sofia that she get some help. "You've changed, love, and while I understand *why* you've changed, you seem so unhappy, and I can't . . . we can't . . . go on like this."

Sofia looked as if she were going to argue with Bailey, but then she started crying. "I know, I know . . . I'm just so mad at everything and everyone! Especially you, and you've been so patient with me."

Bailey put her arms around her, and they hugged for a long time. And then the hug turned into kissing, and then they were on the couch and their clothes were on the floor. They'd barely touched each other since Sofia's diagnosis; in the days and nights before the surgery, they'd had sex often and with a passion even greater than when they'd first gotten together. But then the surgery and radiation had put an end to that, and since then . . . nothing at all until that day.

It isn't unusual for couples to experience a resurgence in their passion for each other in the aftermath of diagnosis but before treatment starts. It may be due to an unspoken need to make memories in the face of potential loss, or it could be an affirmation of love, but many couples describe this time as one of bittersweet desire and pleasure. After treatment though, passion and desire can take a back seat to other intense emotions as well as ongoing side effects of treatment.

That afternoon, despite trying everything, there was no orgasm for either of them. Sofia was shocked, and Bailey was sad that nothing she did worked. Sex with Bailey had always been, in Sofia's words, "spectacular." Bailey had more sexual experience than Sofia, who had come out in her early 20s. Bailey had known she was attracted to women seemingly all her life. And she knew just where and how to touch Sofia to bring her to orgasm. The absence of sex recently had bothered both of them, but they hadn't talked about it, in part because Bailey hadn't wanted to start another argument.

But now they talked about it. Sofia reassured Bailey today's experience was probably a one-time thing—she was upset about what had happened at work. Bailey tried to convince both of them that it was because so much time had passed without sex. But neither of them really believed the idea.

Sofia decided she needed a break from work, and her boss agreed that he could manage for two weeks without her. She'd worked throughout her treatment, other than taking off a week after the lumpectomy. Perhaps her anger had been exacerbated by exhaustion? The break seemed to be helping; she was less irritated with everything and everyone. Bailey had always worked from home—she was a copyeditor for a multinational publishing company—and she liked having Sofia around during the day. The break was also an opportunity for them to see if they could reestablish their sexual relationship. But the problem with Sofia's orgasms persisted.

One morning Sofia had had enough, and she called the women-only clinic she'd attended before the cancer and asked for an appointment with one of the counselors. She had only ever used the clinic for primary care, and she'd seen a nurse practitioner rather than one of the physicians who worked there. She'd never had the need to see a counselor until now, and she was unsure how she was going to talk to a stranger about what was happening. On the day of her appointment, she didn't tell Bailey where she was going or why, and Bailey didn't ask.

Sofia arrived at the clinic slightly out of breath. The clinic was farther from their apartment than she'd remembered, and she'd had to rush to get there on time. Now she tried to relax as she waited for her name to be called.

"Sofia?"

She stood up, and for a moment she considered fleeing. Her discomfort at having to talk about her problem was threatening her desire to get help.

Her name was repeated, this time a little louder.

She walked toward the door being held open by a receptionist and then followed her down a hallway. As she stood in the office, she hoped she didn't have to wait long—her impulse to leave was becoming more urgent.

A few seconds later, an older woman with short gray hair stepped into the room, closing the door behind herself. "Sofia?" The woman's voice was warm but just a little too loud. "I'm Marjorie. Nice to meet you!"

She offered her hand to Sofia, who was then forced to uncross her arms, which she'd been holding against her chest. "Oh, hi. I'm Sofia." She blushed as she realized that Marjorie had just said her name.

"Please, have a seat. Any one of the two chairs will be fine."

Marjorie smiled as she said this, and Sofia noticed two deep dimples in the counselor's cheeks. For some reason, this relaxed her. Marjorie looked like someone in an ad for something comforting, like instant oatmeal.

"What brings you here today?" Marjorie asked.

She didn't have a notebook or clipboard, which helped Sofia feel as if this woman would listen to her fully, rather than concentrate on taking notes. But Sofia wasn't sure to where to start—with her diagnosis or her anger or the sex issue—so she hesitated for a moment. The counselor didn't say anything; she just waited for Sofia to speak.

Then the words poured out of Sofia. And once she'd started to talk, she couldn't stop. Her retelling of what had happened wasn't exactly linear—she started with her taking time off work and ended with the diagnosis. But throughout her story, Marjorie listened, occasionally nodding but not taking her eyes off Sofia's face even for a moment.

"That's a lot," she eventually said when she was sure Sofia had nothing to add. "Let me tell you what I heard, and then you can fill in any details I missed." She repeated Sofia's recitation of what she'd gone through over the previous year. "Did I miss anything?" she asked.

Sofia felt her face turning red. "Um, there's one more thing . . ."

Marjorie could see that Sofia was not comfortable with whatever she had left out.

"Um, there's this issue I'm having . . . I have a great partner, her name is Bailey, and, well, I just can't come anymore . . . and I don't understand why not . . . and . . ." Sofia went on to say she was afraid this was going to affect her relationship with Bailey. She was also worried about the anger thing . . . but felt the lack of orgasms was a more pressing problem.

Marjorie told Sofia that, while the two issues might seem to be separate, in fact they may have been reinforcing each other.

Sofia also explained that she'd been less irritated since taking time off work, and that she and Bailey hadn't argued as often, so perhaps being less stressed and exhausted was helping. "I really want to work on the sex stuff. I think you're right about how that may be making me angry, and if I can fix the anger issue, hopefully it'll also help?"

"One more question, Sofia, if I may?" Marjorie wasn't sure they should be ignoring other issues that may be contributing to Sofia's behavior. "Do you think you're depressed?"

Sofia did not like this question—she'd reacted negatively every time Bailey had asked her the same one. She did not think she was depressed. "No, I am *not* depressed—really, I'm not. I know what depression feels like. I was depressed my first year of college, and this is nothing like that. Please, can we talk about why I came to see you?"

Marjorie didn't respond. She wanted to be client-focused and address what Sofia thought was most important, but on the other hand she didn't want to miss something that could be important. "Can I just ask you a couple of questions, and then we'll move on?"

Sofia nodded—yes, she would answer additional questions if she had to.

Marjorie did a quick assessment for depression (see chapter 7), and Sofia denied experiencing any of its symptoms.

"Okay," Marjorie said, "let's talk about the 'sex stuff,' as you call it. There are a number of reasons why this may be happening, and it's unlikely this has any physical cause. But there could be emotional or psychological reasons for your inability to have an orgasm."

Marjorie explained that, since Sofia was under a lot of stress, she likely had an abundance of stress hormones coursing through her body, and arguing with her partner wasn't helpful.

Sofia felt a wave of guilt flood over herself. She'd been so hard on Bailey, who'd been nothing but supportive and loving to her.

"And another thing," Marjorie said. "In order to be sexually responsive and orgasmic, you need to be present and relaxed during sex. Does that make sense to you?"

Sofia could only nod her head. She'd been anything but relaxed during sex over the past weeks; she was so focused on having an orgasm and thinking about what Bailey was thinking that she'd been in another mental space altogether.

In her book, Emily Nagoski[3] has an entire chapter on the topic of orgasms, including information about what gets in the way of having an orgasm—stress and worry about life and about having an orgasm!—and how to mitigate these obstacles. Importantly, she suggests a focus on pleasure and not on orgasm itself can solve the problem of absent orgasms. While Nagoski talks mostly about heterosexual sex in this particular chapter, she also includes pertinent advice for women in same-sex relationships.

"Orgasm is an act of letting go," continued Marjorie. "Stress about having or not having an orgasm is not going to allow for letting go."

"I guess so," replied Sofia. "But how do I let go? I can't just shut my brain off."

"Let me ask you another question." Marjorie wasn't done asking questions yet. "Why is it so important for you to have an orgasm? Or is it important for your partner?"

"I'm not sure, really . . ." Sofia had never thought about orgasms like this. "I mean, isn't it supposed to be really important for *both* of us?"

"It *can* be important, but it doesn't have to be. Many people are focused on sex as a sensual experience that may or may not include orgasm. Is sex a journey of sensuality and pleasure, or is it goal oriented with orgasm as proof of satisfaction?"

Sofia didn't have an answer to that one, but it left her thinking about talking to Bailey about this whole thing. "So . . . what am I, or rather we, going to do about where we are?" Sofia still wanted to fix the problem.

Marjorie explained that dealing with the absence of orgasms was a process that might take some time. Just as this problem hadn't developed overnight, even though it may seem so, dealing with it would take effort and patience from both Sofia and Bailey.

Sofia replied that she was willing to do the work and have patience—and she hoped Bailey would be on the same page.

"Okay, I'm suggesting that you and your partner do two things," Marjorie said. "The first you can do alone, but including your partner is not a bad idea. Do you have a vibrator?"

Sofia nodded. "Yes, I do, but I haven't used it since I met Bailey . . . There was no need."

"I understand," replied Marjorie, "but I'd like you to dig it out from wherever you put it and use it regularly. You can use it alone or with Bailey, whatever you choose, but the intensity of the vibrations is going to shut out the stress and worry that's in part blocking your orgasms. The sensations can be overwhelming at first, and you may be tempted to stop just before orgasm, or to avoid using it at all. Please persist—using it will allow you to experience pleasure first and foremost, and give you confidence that orgasms are possible once again."

Sofia was listening with great concentration and just a little embarrassment.

"Secondly, I'm going to give you written instructions about something called 'sensate focus' exercises. These are very useful when coupled sex hasn't happened for a while and also in removing the focus from a goal-oriented one to move toward a pleasure- and sensual-oriented activity. I'll explain the process in a minute, but is this something you think you'll find time to engage with? And not just you but your partner too?"

"I'll pretty much do anything within reason to get us back on track!" Of that Sofia was becoming more and more convinced.

Sensate focus exercises (see appendix 2) are an established series of homework exercises that has been used for decades for a variety of sexual problems. While originally developed to help heterosexual couples, the exercises can be modified for same-sex couples where penetration is not the goal. It's important to note that some couples don't go through the linear stages as presented in the original instructions, and you can stop at any stage where you find satisfaction.

Marjorie ended the session by encouraging Sofia to see her with Bailey in a few weeks. She gave Sofia the instructions for the exercises, and they walked out of the office together.

"And you can't ignore the context of where this is happening," Marjorie said. "Stress, irritability, anger, and, yes, even depression that you may not think is part of your context but could be lurking somewhere—these are all part of the picture. And you have to deal with those too!"

Before Sofia turned to leave, she asked whether she could give Marjorie a hug. For the first time in ages, Sofia felt light and hopeful. Maybe, in connecting with Bailey sexually, she could replace some of her anger with a measure of joy. It was about time, she thought as she walked home, preparing what she'd say to Bailey.

CONCLUSION

Despite all the mystery that surrounds orgasm, it's a matter of genital sensations being interpreted by the brain as pleasurable, and then messages from the brain traveling to the pelvic muscles, which contract and produce most of the sensations of orgasm. The pleasure centers of the brain light up to further enhance the feelings

There are many possible reasons why someone isn't able to have an orgasm, including physical or emotional causes. Loss of orgasms, in medical terms "anorgasmia," is not something that's well understood or researched, but it causes distress for both the survivor and their partner. Finding a solution is more important than the cause in many instances.

TAKEAWAYS

- An orgasm is not necessary for sexual satisfaction, but for many, it is the goal of sexual activity.

- In men, orgasm is usually accompanied by ejaculation of semen, but this doesn't always happen. Ejaculation is important if the couple want to conceive, and for some men, the sensation of semen moving through the urethra may provide additional sensation.

- Alterations in the sensation of or a complete absence of orgasm is distressing for many, and it's often not discussed with health-care providers or even a partner!

- While there may be a physical reason for a lack of orgasm, the emotional aspects are important to consider and may contribute to a self-fulfilling reaction, with anxiety about having an orgasm preventing the orgasm itself.

- Being in the moment and staying relaxed are key elements in having an orgasm; feeling angry or stressed gets in the way of these elements.

- The more a person focuses on having an orgasm, the less likely it is to happen!

RECOMMENDED READING

For further reading, I recommend the following books:

The Science of Orgasm, by Barry R. Komisaruk, Carlos Beyer-Flores, and Beverly Whipple

Come as You Are, by Emily Nagoski

WEBSITES FOR ADDITIONAL INFORMATION

American Cancer Society
https://www.cancer.org/cancer/managing-cancer/side -effects/fertility-and-sexual-side-effects/sexuality-for -women-with-cancer/cancer-sex-sexuality.html

Leukemia and Lymphoma Society (YouTube video)
https://www.lls.org/patient-education-webcasts /sexuality-young-adult-cancer-what-you-need-know

Livestrong
https://livestrong.org/resources/male-sexual-health -after-cancer/

National Cancer Institute (NIH)
https://www.cancer.gov/about-cancer/treatment/side -effects/sexuality-men

CHAPTER 6

"It hurts—why is this happening?"

Pain with Sex

After cancer treatment, some people experience pain when they attempt any form of sexual touch or activity. It can be devastating when something that was once a source of pleasure becomes something to fear and even avoid. Among men treated for prostate cancer with radiation therapy, 15% reported painful orgasms.[1,2] But sexual pain can occur at any point during sexual activity. In women, attempted penetration often causes tightening or spasm of the pelvic-floor muscles as the body responds to pain; up to 65% of women report this kind of pain.[3] In addition, women may also experience pain during orgasm as the pelvic-floor muscles contract.

WILL AND JONATHAN

Will and Jonathan, both 35 years old, met at the gym 3 years ago. They had friends in common, so it was strange they'd never met before. They even lived near each other and went to the same grocery store, but their paths had never crossed before that day in the locker room. It was attraction at first sight; they started talking, then they went for a drink at a nearby bar that evening, and they kept talking until the bar closed down for the night. Will was an elementary school teacher, and Jonathan was a librarian at a liberal arts college.

Four months ago, Will was diagnosed with testicular cancer. It had all started with a swollen testicle that he'd assumed was due to his workout, which had changed when he'd started working with a personal trainer. He and Jonathan had a healthy competition over which of them was more "jacked." Will had seemed to be losing the competition, so he'd engaged a personal trainer, who'd switched up his weight routine. It was after that change when he'd noticed one testicle was swollen and a little painful. He'd ignored it initially, but Jonathan insisted he get it checked out.

Will went to an urgent care clinic because he didn't have a primary care provider. He saw a nurse practitioner, whose face gave away his concern when he examined Will. Something was wrong, and the conclusion so far was that it was not likely a gym injury. Within a week Will saw a urologist, and a week later he had surgery to remove the testicle. He had a prosthetic testicle inserted at the time of the surgery; the urologist had recommended this, and he'd agreed.

While not necessary, men may opt to have a testicular prosthetic inserted in the scrotum so there's no visible sign of the missing testicle. This may help men maintain their masculine self-image.

The recovery period was painful, more painful than Will had been told it might be, but after two weeks he felt well enough to go back to work. He had a follow-up appointment with the urologist a month later, and he was relieved to learn he wouldn't need any additional treatment. He was eager to get back to the gym, but Jonathan persuaded him to wait the full six weeks as instructed. This was not easy; Will was concerned he'd lose muscle mass and put on weight. His appearance was important to him, and the thought of Jonathan alone at the gym with all the other attractive men made him feel insecure. Not working out also deprived him of some much-needed relief from the frustration he often felt after a day of teaching grade 5 students, who could be challenging. He found he was counting the days until he could go back to his personal trainer and weight lifting.

But there was another source of frustration for him, one that grew out of his relationship with Jonathan. The day after Will had seen the urologist for his follow-up, he suggested to Jonathan that they should resume having sex. A month was a long time to go without it, and he was buoyed by the news that he didn't need further treatment. How better to celebrate the all clear from the surgery? But Jonathan wasn't so sure this was a good idea; was it safe for Will after the surgery? He asked Will whether the urologist had said anything about that—and if he hadn't, why had Will not asked? Will just shrugged and replied that if the issue was important, the urologist would have said something.

Sex is often not discussed between health-care providers and patients,[4] even when the health-care provider is a urologist or gynecologist, who should be able to talk about such things! The usual convention is that you should avoid sex for six weeks after surgery to sexual organs (and after other surgeries as well), but there is no clear evidence for this specific amount of time. It's important to ask your health-care provider about how long you should avoid sex, among other physical activities, especially if they don't take the lead and offer the information.

Will was a little hurt that Jonathan didn't seem interested in doing anything sexual for another couple of weeks. Their sex life had been great until his diagnosis and surgery, and he'd assumed they would pick up where they'd left off. But Jonathan didn't seem interested, and Will wasn't sure why. He went back to the gym exactly six weeks after the surgery. His personal trainer explained to him that he needed to take things slowly and that he needed to be patient. Will was prepared to be patient about his workouts, but his patience was running out with Jonathan!

The next weekend Will decided he needed to do something about the situation. He waited for the right opportunity, and it came on Sunday morning as they were walking home after their workout.

"Jon, we need to talk."

"Okay, what about? Is something wrong?"

Will felt his frustration building up, and he took a deep breath before responding. "Yes, there is something wrong, something really wrong! We haven't had sex in over six weeks, and you don't seem to mind!"

Jonathan stopped walking in the middle of the sidewalk and almost got bumped into by a jogger right behind them. "Of course I mind!" he replied. "Don't you think I've missed it? Missed you? But I don't want you to damage something . . ."

"You—I mean we—can't damage anything! If it's okay for me to work out, then it must be okay to have sex, don't you think?"

"I don't know what to think, Will. You didn't get any information, and I'm just scared, you know?"

"Well, I'm not scared, Jon. Not even one little bit, and while it's really sweet that you're worried about me, you don't need to be!"

The conversation seemed to have persuaded Jon, because they walked the last few blocks to their apartment faster than usual. They showered together even though the small shower stall was a tight fit for them both at the same time. Then they were in such a rush that they didn't bother drying off; they fell onto their king-size bed, leaving a trail of water from the bathroom to the bedroom.

The sex was okay—just okay—but neither of them said anything about it. Jonathan didn't notice when Will grimaced as he rolled over to put on his glasses. Will didn't say anything to Jonathan, who dozed off as he usually did after sex.

Will lay next to him for a few minutes then started to get up to go shower again. He was barely six inches off the bed when a wave of pain made him sit down quickly, almost missing the edge of the mattress. What was this? He sat for a few minutes, Jonathan's soft breathing the only sound in the room. The pain lessened as he sat there, but as soon as he moved, it came back. Will managed to reach backward and tap Jonathan on the arm.

"What? What is it? You want to go again?" Jonathan mumbled happily.

"Jon, wake up! Something's wrong."

Jonathan sat up immediately as Will bent over, one arm wrapped around his body. "What happened?" Jonathan's voice was loud. "Are you okay? Stupid question, you're not okay. What is it?"

"I don't know . . . It's just pain . . . like my whole body is spasming."

Will must've sounded distressed because Jonathan reached for his phone to call 911.

"No, don't do that!" His voice came out shrill. "I think it's passing now. Just hang on a bit . . . maybe it'll go away . . ." Will slowly straightened up, his breathing shallow. He felt weak and sweaty.

Jonathan moved to his side and slowly helped him to the shower. As Will stood under the water, Jonathan waited and watched. The pain lessened, and within 10 minutes Will felt better.

"We're going to the urgent care clinic right now!" Jonathan was insistent, and Will didn't argue; something wasn't right, and he did not want to experience pain like that again.

At the clinic, Will was happy to be brought into a room with the same nurse practitioner he'd seen before. But he was surprised when Jonathan greeted him by name.

"Adam! Hi! I didn't know you worked here. Will, this is Adam. I've known him for ages, but we lost touch. What a surprise!"

Will had wondered if the nurse practitioner was gay, and Jonathan knowing him seemed to confirm it, which lessened his current embarrassment a little.

Adam smiled at Will. "Will, I'm not going to say it's nice to see you again because there's a reason you're here. How can I help you?"

Will started to explain what had occurred, but Jonathan interrupted him. "Do you want me to leave the room?"

Will shook his head and briefly described to Adam what he'd experienced. The nurse practitioner listened carefully and then asked some questions that Will answered.

Yes, he had been working out, and, yes, he was using fairly heavy weights at the gym. No, he had not had any pain while at the gym, but he had felt a heaviness in his pelvis over the last few days.

Jonathan looked a little irritated when Will admitted this. Will knew he should've told Jonathan about it. He didn't say anything now and waited for Adam to speak.

"This sounds like a pelvic-floor issue to me." The nurse practitioner sounded confident in his assessment. "I'd like you to see a pelvic-floor physiotherapist for a thorough examination. You may have started with weights a little too soon, or used weights that are too heavy."

Jonathan looked at Will, who avoided eye contact. Will didn't want to see the smug look Jonathan probably had on his face.

"Can I see the physiotherapist who works at the gym we go to?" Will asked.

"It's better that you see a physiotherapist who is an expert in the pelvic floor," Adam responded. "Most physiotherapists don't specialize in this area and so aren't that helpful in cases such as yours. There's a really good person that I refer to. Her practice is fairly close, and she usually makes time to fit in anyone I refer to her. Can I go ahead and make that happen?"

Will responded quickly. "Sure, go ahead."

The pelvic floor comprises pairs of muscles that support the bladder, urethra, and bowels, and in women the vagina and uterus as well. These muscles lie like a sling from the pubic bone in the front to the tailbone (sacrum) in the back. A pelvic-floor physiotherapist is a specialist in assessing and treating pelvic-floor problems using a variety of techniques. These include manual therapy, biofeedback, electrical stimulation, and exercises to do at home.

Will was a bit disappointed that he had to have an appointment with someone else and that the physiotherapist was a woman. Was this going to be embarrassing, he wondered. He got up to leave, wincing as he rose from the chair. Adam and Jonathan were talking as they all left the exam room and walked through the waiting room, and neither noticed that he was still in pain.

By the time Will and Jonathan got back to their apartment, the physiotherapist, whose name was Kelli, had left a message on Will's phone with an appointment for the next Wednesday. Jonathan asked whether Will wanted him to go with him to the appointment, but Will refused. Jonathan had to take unpaid leave to attend appointments with him, and he'd already taken off time after Will's surgery. This had dented his take-home pay, and their emergency savings had suffered.

Will was apprehensive about the appointment and was glad he didn't have long to wait to see Kelli. At the appointment, her broad smile and firm handshake put him at ease. She asked him a lot of questions before doing the physical assessment. Even though the examination itself was uncomfortable, both physically and emotionally, she was professional, which helped. He was a little surprised that he was only a tiny bit embarrassed, even though she was a woman and the exam was invasive.

A proper examination of the pelvic floor requires an internal examination. This is done through the rectum in men and vagina in women. Some physiotherapists will also use an ultrasound on the perineum (the area between the scrotum in men, and the opening of the vagina in women, and the anus). While many people may find this embarrassing, remember the physiotherapist is a professional. They'll drape the lower half of your body and do their best to put you at ease by explaining exactly what they're going to do and asking for your consent for any physical touch.

After the exam, Kelli described her observations. "Those muscles of yours were really tight, I would say in spasm, during my examination," she said. "I'm sorry if this caused you pain, but it's necessary to get an accurate picture of what's going on."

Will took a deep breath; he had been holding his breath during the exam despite the physiotherapist encouraging him to relax. He felt bad that he hadn't answered the physiotherapist honestly when she'd asked him about when he'd experienced pain. He had told her he'd felt pain at the gym, which wasn't true, and he'd left out the acute pain he'd had with orgasm.

Contractions of the pelvic-floor muscles contribute to the sensation of orgasm, as explained in chapter 5. If the muscles are tight or in spasm, this is termed "hypertonic," and if the muscles are too loose, they're called "hypotonic." Both situations affect the sensations of orgasm. If the muscles are hypertonic, orgasm can be painful, and if the muscles are hypotonic, orgasm can be absent or the sensations diminished.

Kelli sensed there was more to Will's story; she had treated a lot of people with a history of cancer, especially those with cancer involving the pelvic area, and she knew cancer treatment often led to pelvic-floor and sexual problems. "A hypertonic pelvic floor often leads to painful orgasms. Is everything okay in that department?"

Will blushed as he admitted that pain with sex, specifically orgasm, was what had led him to seek medical care.

"Okay, let's talk about solutions," Kelly said. "We can approach this in two ways. The first is for you to learn how to relax the pelvic-floor muscles. The second is finding if there are any trigger points in the muscles and massaging them to release the tension in the muscle fibers. This is going to take time, but it's also going to be worth it. Does this sound like something you're prepared to work on?"

"Yes, of course I want to fix this. When can I, rather we, start?"

"If it's okay with you, I think we can start today, with me showing you where the trigger points are in those muscles. I felt three or four, but I'm going to have to insert my finger again to do that. Sorry about that, but it's the only way . . ."

Kelli explained that he was going to need regular massages of the muscles to release the trigger points, so they were going to see a lot of each other if he was willing to continue the treatment.

Will was not really happy about that, but he was also not happy about having pain with an orgasm. "Short term pain for longer gain, I guess!" He tried to make a joke of it, and Kelli smiled.

"I'll be gentle, I promise," she said. "And after I've done a short massage, I'll explain how to do the exercises to relax those muscles. It's important for me to be able to feel how effectively you can relax the muscles, and that way you also know that you're doing them correctly. Is it okay to start now?"

Will sighed and nodded. He wondered how he was going to tell Jonathan about this; it was going to make for interesting after-dinner conversation.

After hearing about what the appointment had involved, Jonathan was pleased that Will had refused his offer to go with him to the physiotherapist; it sounded like a very private issue. But . . . "Is there some way I can help with, um . . . home exercises?"

Will swatted his arm. "No way!" But he laughed as he said it.

He had a follow-up appointment set with Kelli the next week, so he was diligent about doing the pelvic-floor-muscle exercises. She'd suggested doing them three times a day, and in order to remember to do them, he'd decided to link them to mealtimes. Every day as he prepared his breakfast and lunch, and then just before they sat down for dinner, Will performed them—until within the week, doing the exercises had become routine.

He was excited to see Kelli again to learn whether there was any difference in the tone of the muscles. And there was! While not yet perfect, or as perfect as they were ever going to be, Kelli congratulated him on his progress. He couldn't wait to get home to see if an orgasm would feel better; he hoped Jonathan could leave work early!

LUCY AND RALPH

Lucy knew something was wrong when she experienced vaginal bleeding years after she'd gone through menopause. At 66 years old, she instinctively knew this was not normal. She made an urgent appointment with her gynecologist, who performed an endometrial (lining of the uterus) biopsy. The news was not good; Lucy had endometrial cancer. The diagnosis brought up a whole host of memories of her mother, who'd died from ovarian cancer when Lucy had been in her early 20s. Her husband of 45 years, Ralph, tried his best to comfort her, but Lucy was consumed by fear that her fate was going to be that of her mother's. Her gynecologist, Dr. Brooks, tried to reassure Lucy that endometrial cancer was not the same as ovarian cancer and that treatments for cancer had evolved over the 40 years since her mother's diagnosis and early death. Lucy insisted that if she were to have surgery to remove her uterus then they needed to remove her ovaries as well. Dr. Brooks agreed and referred her to a radiation oncologist to see if she needed radiation too. Lucy was not going to take no for an answer, and when she met with the radiation oncologist one week after her surgery, she was happy to hear she would have two kinds of radiation—external beam radiation and internal radiation. The nurse who worked with the radiation oncologist described a long list of potential side effects from the radiation, but Lucy barely listened; she wanted any and all treatments to destroy the cancer, and she would deal with the side effects later.

Recovery from the surgery hadn't been too bad, but the radiation was a different matter. Lucy had skin damage on her lower abdomen from the external radiation that looked and felt like a severe sunburn. She had the fair skin that often goes along with being a redhead, and she'd never exposed the skin on her abdomen to the sun. She also had a lot of pain deep in her pelvis; the radiation oncologist told her that it was likely because she had tissue damage at the top of her vagina from the internal radiation. He said that it would heal with time and that an internal examination was not advisable as it would only cause more damage.

Lucy and Ralph hadn't had children, and while their infertility had been devastating when they'd learned about it, she now felt comforted that she had no female children who would experience cancer like her mother and now her. Even though her gynecologist had explained there was no genetic risk of passing on her cancer, she still somehow felt better. She and Ralph had enjoyed many years of travel, and they had nephews and nieces, and a couple of great-nephews, whom they'd loved to spoil over the years.

As the radiation oncologist had predicted, Lucy felt better as time passed. The internal pain was completely resolved as was her fatigue. The diagnosis had spurred her to make some lifestyle changes; as her energy levels increased, she started a daily regimen of walking, and she tried to cut back on the amount of red meat they ate. Ralph went along with the changes, and he looked as if he'd lost a few pounds. Their daily walks usually ended up at a nearby coffee bar, where they soon found a group of like-minded people, who became new friends.

"A silver lining, you could call it," was how Ralph described the experience.

After almost three months, the new routine was now normal for the couple, and life settled down. Lucy didn't need any additional treatment, and her gynecologist and radiation oncologist had given her the all clear she had desperately hoped for. The daily walks with Ralph allowed them to talk about future travel plans, and they booked a cruise for Ralph's birthday at the end of the year.

The only thing missing was sex. Things had slowed down when Lucy had gone through menopause; and of course, while she been in treatment, sex hadn't been an option. Ralph had never been a touchy-feely kind of man, and their twice-a-month sex date had been the primary way they'd connected physically. Lucy missed the physical contact, but she had long ago accepted that hand-holding or hugs were not part of their relationship. He was a good man, and he always told her he loved her before they went to sleep, so that was that.

Physical touch leads to the production of oxytocin, the so-called bonding hormone. Touch isn't vital for emotional connection in relationships, but for some the absence of touch results in something described as "skin hunger." The opposite of this is what many parents of young children, particularly mothers, describe as being "touched out" by the constant physical contact with their babies or young children.

The next three months before the cruise flew by. In the days before they left, Lucy was so excited that she almost forgot to buy a birthday card for Ralph. She remembered to get one the day before their flight to meet the ship, and she managed to find one at the grocery store. But she didn't have time to buy him a gift.

"Well, I've given him a birthday gift for the past 45 years, so maybe he'll forgive me this one time!" she thought. She made a mental note to make up for this by giving him the one thing that had been missing for the previous six months. They would have sex on his birthday on the ship, so she packed a fancy nightgown that had been pushed to the back of a drawer since his last birthday. That had become a long-running joke between them—the nightgown only appeared on special occasions like birthdays, anniversaries, and New Year's Eve.

Ralph's birthday was on the third day of the weeklong cruise. That night, they had a lovely dinner with a bottle of sparkling wine, followed by ice-cream cake with a single candle. The servers in the dining room sang happy birthday to him as he blushed and smiled. At Lucy's insistence, they passed on the evening's entertainment and went back to their cabin. Lucy went into the en suite bathroom, closing the door behind her; this alerted Ralph to the possibility that something else was on the agenda for the evening, and he undressed quickly and got into bed. Lucy appeared shortly after that in the "special" nightgown. She too had lost weight, and for the first time in a long while, she felt confident in her body.

But her feelings of confidence did not last long. They were both in a hurry, which might have been due to excitement after the long absence or some apprehension about what sex would be like after Lucy's treatment. Or perhaps their rushing was because of something else entirely, but as soon as Ralph entered her, she let out a yelp of pain. Ralph immediately moved off her, his face reflecting shock and concern. Lucy rolled over and almost fell off the bed; she hurried to the bathroom, not bothering to shut the door behind her.

External and internal radiation to the pelvis to treat gynecologic cancer causes the vagina to narrow and tighten. In addition, as part of the surgery to remove the uterus, the upper third of the vagina that surrounds the cervix is also removed. Tissue damage inside the vagina from the radiation also alters the elasticity of the vaginal walls. All of this results in pain with penetration.

Ralph followed Lucy and stopped at the bathroom door. She was sitting on the closed toilet, doubled over, tears running down her face.

"What happened? Are you okay? What did I do?" His voice was soft with concern.

"I don't know . . . it just hurt so bad . . ." Lucy wiped the tears from her face as the nurse's words came back to her. "The radiation nurse said something about shortening of my vagina, but she didn't mention that it would hurt so bad."

Ralph didn't know what to say. He'd offered to go with his wife to all of her appointments, but Lucy had refused. He'd grown used to her fierce independence over the years, but now he wished he had been more insistent and pushed back about going with her to her treatments. What information had he missed? As he watched her get up slowly, one hand cradling her lower abdomen, he tried to think of something to say. All he knew was that it was probably better to say nothing, so he kept quiet.

At various times before and during cancer treatment, patients are given information about side effects and how to manage them. It's common for people not to review or retain this information, and so when side effects do occur, they often come as a shock. There are solutions to this; first, health-care providers should talk about these details on more than one occasion. Before treatment starts, patients can forget information because they're anxious. Second, it's important for the patient to have a trusted family member or friend with them to take notes or listen carefully to the information provided—four ears are better than two! And third, verbal communication should be followed up with written material about where to find additional information.

It took a while for Lucy and Ralph to fall asleep. They woke late the next morning, and they both acted as if nothing had happened the night before. For the rest of the cruise, they ignored that evening, and when Lucy packed her bag the night before they disembarked, she left her nightgown in the back of a drawer on purpose. On the flight home, they were both deep in thought. Ralph wasn't sure what to say or do, and Lucy made mental notes about who to call for help. She didn't have any follow-up appointments with the radiation oncologist, but she was due to see her gynecologist the week after they returned; she would start there.

Dr. Brooks listened carefully as Lucy told her what had happened. She nodded every now and then as Lucy described the pain—like being torn apart—and her face showed she empathized with her patient's experience.

"I suspect that if you allow me to examine you, I'll be able to confirm that your vagina has been damaged by both the surgery and the radiation. Is that something you want me to do, or should we assume there is damage and talk about what can be done about that?"

"I really don't want anyone or anything to go 'down there,'" Lucy admitted. "I just can't bear the thought of going through the pain again."

"Okay, that's fine," replied the physician. "I do have one question—did no one talk to you about using dilators after the radiation?" She tried to keep her tone neutral; she didn't want her patient to feel she was being blamed.

"I honestly can't remember," Lucy said. "It was all a blur at that time. Maybe the nurse did tell me about that, but I must have forgotten or just ignored her. It's all my fault . . . and now it's too late . . ." Lucy was close to tears. She felt guilty and afraid that this was her fault and nothing could be done. Was this the end of sex forever? Even though for the last few years their sex life had been nowhere near what it had once been, it was still enjoyable.

"I don't think it's too late, Lucy." Dr Brooks spoke softly. "It's just over three or four months since the end of treatment, and I have some suggestions that I hope will help. I'm going to show you how to use a dilator and also prescribe some local estrogen cream to be used with the dilator. This is not something that will be fixed overnight, but with patience and consistent use, I have every hope that you'll see improvement."

Women who have been treated for gynecologic or rectal/anal cancer should be encouraged to use vaginal dilators on a regular basis to help keep the vagina open after radiation therapy. A dilator is a device, usually made of plastic or silicone, that's inserted into the vagina. The radiation oncologist may prescribe a dilator with a certain circumference, or the radiation therapy department may provide one. Using estrogen cream as a lubricant when inserting the dilator is also helpful to keep the tissues flexible.

The next time Lucy saw the gynecologist, she reported that she'd used the dilator she'd gotten, as well as the estrogen cream. When Dr. Brooks examined her, she remarked that the tissues looked healthy even though her vagina was shorter than before and that using the dilator wouldn't change this. She explained to Lucy that because her vagina was now shorter, penetration during sexual intercourse could cause pressure at the top of the vagina (called the "vaginal vault") or even pain.

"And how is your sex life these days, Lucy? Are things better after using the dilator?"

Lucy shook her head. "I've been too scared to try anything," she admitted. "My husband hasn't suggested we try, and frankly, it's just not something we've ever talked about. Before this, we didn't need to, you know? And now it's just too hard."

"I hear you. But are both of you okay with not having sex?"

"I guess so . . ." Lucy hesitated. The truth was that there was a distance between them, and there were times when she felt they would never again have the close feeling that had once existed. "But what can I do about this? I've been using the dilator and the cream . . . but what if we try and sex hurts?"

"Well, you won't know until you try," the doctor said. "But you have to talk to your husband about this before you try. You need to take things slowly. You need to be aroused before penetration, and you need to use a good lubricant. I have some samples I can give you, but communication is still very important. I'm here to help, and I can refer you to a sex therapist if you need help with communicating."

"Oh, I don't think we need a therapist!" Lucy wasn't ready for that yet; talking so openly to her gynecologist was challenging enough!

She went home, and while Dr. Brooks's words were still in her ears, she repeated to Ralph what she had suggested. Ralph was more than eager to try something, anything, so that evening they tried. They took it slow, and they used one of the lubricants, but it still hurt. Maybe not as bad as on the ship, and this time the pain was deeper, as if his penis were bumping against something. Lucy gritted her teeth and got through it, but it was not pleasurable, and she was glad when it was over. Ralph fell asleep immediately, a small smile on his face.

Lucy called her gynecologist as soon as the clinic opened. She told her what had happened, forcing the words out while trying to hide her sadness.

"Ah, I thought this might happen," Dr. Brooks said. "There is a potential solution to this as well, if you're willing to try it."

"I'll pretty much try anything at this point," Lucy said.

Dr. Brooks explained that, because Lucy's vagina was now shorter, her husband's penis was bumping against the top of her vagina (the vaginal vault), which caused the pain. "One of the strategies that may help is if the woman is on top during intercourse. You can then control the depth of thrusting. Other sexual positions can also be tried—side lying for example. There is also something called the Ohnut, which acts as a buffer to deep penetration when placed over the erect penis. I have samples of these, and if you and your husband want to come in to my office, I can show both of you what they look and feel like."

The Ohnut is a soft, flexible series of up to four stackable rings worn externally by the man at the base of the penis. It can be used with both silicone- and water-based lubricants, and it acts like a shock absorber, preventing penetration that's too deep and causes pain for the woman.

"Oh, I don't know if Ralph will want to try that or even if he wants to talk about it!" Lucy wasn't sure whether she could even raise the topic with her husband.

"How about I send you some information about this in the mail? I have a pamphlet that describes the device and has images of the Ohnut as well. You may be surprised at his response—I imagine he isn't happy about causing you pain."

Lucy considered this for a moment. Maybe Ralph would be interested. It was worth a try. "Okay, please send that to me . . . and thank you."

Lucy was still not convinced, but if the rings solved the problem they were having, trying them would be worth this awkwardness, wouldn't it? To her surprise, when she showed the pamphlet to Ralph, he seemed interested—in fact, he was very interested. His enthusiasm for trying the device made her think he wasn't willing to give up on their sex life. And while she was nervous, she was also excited because perhaps, maybe, their sex life wasn't over at all.

CONCLUSION

Pain with or after sex is not normal and should not be ignored. Even though it may feel embarrassing to explain what you're experiencing, even to a health-care provider, this isn't something you should disregard; there may be a simple explanation, or the pain may need further investigation. Pelvic-floor physiotherapists have specialized and intensive training in assessing the muscles of the pelvic floor and treating conditions associated with these muscles. These conditions include problems with urination and bowel movements, as well as sexual problems. The American Physical Therapy Association has a special division, the Academy of Pelvic Health Physical Therapy, that offers resources about this specialized practice and a link to find locations of pelvic-floor physiotherapists across the United States. You can find the academy at https://www.aptapelvichealth.org.

TAKEAWAYS

- Pain during or after sex is not normal and should not be ignored.

- There are many reasons why you might experience pain with sex, including loss of lubrication for women, internal scarring from cancer surgery, or fear of pain itself.

- In women, pain with sexual touch or penetration often causes the muscles of the pelvic floor to contract, causing further pain.

- In men who have had surgery or radiation to the pelvis, internal scarring or damage to the muscles of the pelvic floor may result in pain with orgasm.

- A tight pelvic floor, caused by using incorrect technique while doing pelvic-floor exercises or doing these exercises too often, is also a cause of pain with penetration or pain with orgasm.

- While you might be embarrassed to talk about your pain, even with a health-care provider, it's important to try to find the cause and to identify solutions that may help.

- Ignoring the problem or hiding it from your partner doesn't make it disappear. Your partner will most likely be upset if they find out later they've caused you pain. Open and honest communication is a vital part of finding solutions to any sexual problem.

WEBSITES FOR ADDITIONAL INFORMATION

Academy of Pelvic Health Physical Therapy
https://www.aptapelvichealth.org

Mayo Clinic
https://www.mayoclinic.org/diseases-conditions
/painful-intercourse/symptoms-causes/syc-20375967

National Cancer Institute (NIH)
https://www.cancer.gov/about-cancer/treatment/side
-effects/sexuality-men

OncoLink
https://www.oncolink.org/support/sexuality-fertility
/sexuality/vaginal-dryness-and-painful-intercourse

CHAPTER 7

"My world is gray—I hate this feeling"

Depression and Anxiety

Many couples experience changes in their sex life after cancer. They may go through a range of emotions, including anxiety and depression due to the multiple losses they face during and after treatment. Depression is common after a diagnosis of cancer; up to 66% of women with breast cancer[1] and 25% with gynecologic cancer[2] experience this. Approximately 12% of men diagnosed report depression[3]—the lower percentage likely reflects the better prognosis of the most common cancer in men, prostate cancer. Rates of anxiety are slightly lower in these groups, with 33% of women with breast cancer[1] and 27% with gynecologic cancer[2] experiencing the condition. Among men with prostate cancer, 23% report anxiety.[3]

Depression and anxiety may occur together, but they don't always; a qualified health-care provider will be able to identify whether you're experiencing these two conditions. This chapter describes the struggles of two couples as they try to adapt to the changes in their relationship.

LIONEL AND RUBY

No man wants to hear the words "You have penile cancer," no matter his age or relationship status. But this is what Lionel heard when he saw his family physician one week after he had a biopsy of white patches on the skin of his penis. He hadn't been aware of the presence of the patches; he hardly looked at that part of his anatomy these days, mostly because his large stomach made it difficult. And it had been some time since his wife, Ruby, had paid any attention to that area too. His family physician, Dr. Bergen, had noticed them at Lionel's annual checkup and had taken a small sample to send it to be examined.

"Cancer? On my penis? How does that happen?" Lionel had never heard of anyone with this kind of cancer.

Penile cancer is a type of cancer that usually starts on the skin of the penis. If not found and treated early, the cancer can grow into the deeper layers of the organ, leading to the need for more aggressive treatment, including surgery to remove part of or the entire organ (this is called a "penectomy"). Some penile cancers are linked to the human papilloma virus (HPV), which can cause cervical cancer in women as well as head and neck cancer. Risk factors include a history of smoking.

Dr. Bergen explained these details to Lionel, who was barely listening. He shook his head when the physician asked whether he had any questions. He wanted to go home, but that meant having to tell Ruby. How was he going to tell her? She tended to cry at the drop of a hat, and then he had to comfort her—but what he needed most was for her to comfort him.

Lionel managed to find his car in the parking garage, then make his way to their house, which was 30 minutes from the doctor's office. On the drive, he was startled once or twice by a car honking behind him at a traffic light; in a daze, he hadn't noticed the light had turned green.

Ruby was in the garden when he pulled into the driveway. She waved at him and went back to pruning the roses, her favorite pastime. Lionel sat in the car for a few minutes, his thoughts scattered as he tried to find the words that would shatter her life.

Ruby came over to the car when she noticed that he hadn't gotten out. "Lionel, honey, is something wrong? Are you feeling okay?"

Lionel realized he couldn't avoid telling her what Dr. Bergen had said. He hadn't told his wife about the biopsy, and now he was not sure why he'd hidden that from her. "It's cancer!" The words just burst out of his mouth, and he watched silently as Ruby's mouth opened and shut without a sound, and her eyes filled with tears.

"What do you mean?" she finally managed to say.

"He said it was cancer of my . . . you know . . . my . . ." Now Lionel was struggling to find words. "It's my penis!" he managed to blurt out.

"Your what?" Ruby seemed not sure she'd heard right.

Lionel got out of the car slowly. He started to walk toward the house, motioning for Ruby to follow. Once they were inside, he sat down on a kitchen chair. His body seemed disconnected from his brain, and he felt every one of his 70 years. He told her what he could remember about the appointment, which was barely anything, and she immediately went to the phone and called Dr. Bergen's office—she wanted to make an appointment to hear what all this meant. She was no longer crying and had gone into crisis mode, as she always had when their children were young and had hurt themselves.

"Dr. Bergen is going to see us at 4:30 tomorrow afternoon. And you're going to do exactly what he tells you to do. And you're not going to hide anything from me ever again. And after we hear what you have to do, we're going to talk to the children."

Her firmness was reassuring to Lionel, and he did exactly what she said. The next day, they met with Dr. Bergen, who explained that Lionel was going to need to see someone called a "uro-oncologist," a urologist whose specialty was cancer of the urinary system. Lionel would likely need additional tests before a treatment plan was made.

The next few weeks were filled with doctors' appointments and tests, all of which were embarrassing since the focus was on a part of his body that was so private. And most of the health-care providers looked so young—and some of them were women!

What no one asked about, and what Ruby didn't seem to notice, was that Lionel was becoming more and more withdrawn every day. He had no appetite, and even though he was tired, so tired, he woke frequently at night. He didn't want to disturb Ruby, so he spent most of the night on the couch in the den; she didn't seem to mind, and they didn't talk about it.

After all the tests were completed, they met with the uro-oncologist, who told them Lionel needed to have surgery to remove part of his penis. This was shocking; neither of them had even thought this was a possibility.

"Is there no other choice of treatment?" Ruby once again moved into crisis mode.

"I'm afraid the cancer was deeper in the tissues of the penis than we had hoped," the doctor replied. "Your husband has a better chance of cure if we do this."

"Then that is what he's going to do!" Ruby said. "When can you schedule the operation?"

Lionel sat quietly as Ruby and the urologist talked. With Ruby in charge, Lionel felt relieved, and he could pretend the conversation going on around him was about someone else.

Lionel's withdrawn response is common; a feeling of discon-nection from what's being talked about is a protective response to life-altering news. At any appointment, especially when treatment plans are being discussed, it's important to have someone with you who can listen, absorb the information, and take notes. Some health-care providers will allow you to record these discussions so you can review the information later; per-mission to record the discussion is necessary. While having someone take notes is an alternative, the notetaker may not be able to listen and write at the same time, and they might miss some information.

Lionel did exactly what he was told to do. He had the sur-gery, and about one inch of his penis was removed, leaving the rest intact. While the uro-oncologist was happy with the re-sults, Lionel could barely bring himself to look at that area of his body. He had a urinary catheter in place to drain his blad-der while he recovered, and it was not comfortable at all. He didn't mention this to Ruby because he didn't want her to look at that part of him either. She emptied the catheter bag, and that was bad enough.

He went to see Dr. Bergen to have the catheter removed, and when the physician entered the room, Lionel asked Ruby to leave. She understood why, but she was worried about what in-formation she'd miss while she was gone.

Fortunately, Dr. Bergen understood the situation, and as soon as Lionel was dressed and sitting in a chair, he invited Ruby to come back into the room.

"Lionel, this surgery can have a huge impact on the man's emotions," the doctor said. "Have you noticed any changes in your mood? Ruby, have you noticed anything?"

Ruby shook her head; she'd been so busy taking care of her husband, emptying the catheter bag and keeping track of his pain medications, that she hadn't really paid attention to his moods. Plus, she was trying to manage her own emotions and the fear of losing her husband.

Lionel didn't say anything. The truth was that he was feeling down for the first time in his life, but he didn't have the words to explain it.

"I'm going to ask you a couple of questions if that's okay," Dr. Bergen said.

"Sure," Lionel replied.

"Over the last two weeks, how often have you been bothered by a lack of interest or pleasure in doing things?"

Lionel hesitated. "Almost every day," he said.

"And what about feeling hopeless, depressed, or down?"

"The same . . . most days."

These two questions are a screening tool for depression known as the "Patient Health Questionnaire," or PHQ-2.[4] There are other screening tools for depression that are used to identify people who may need further assessment. If needed, the health-care provider can then use further tools and clinical assessment to make the diagnosis and offer treatment.

Ruby was shocked and ashamed that she hadn't noticed Lionel was feeling so down. She reached out to hold his hand, but he barely noticed.

Dr. Bergen asked more questions about how Lionel was sleeping, whether his appetite had changed, what his energy level was like, whether his movement or speech seemed to have slowed, and whether he had difficulty concentrating, felt bad about himself, or thought about hurting himself or that he was better off dead. Lionel answered that he wasn't sleeping well and often felt tired, and he generally felt sad. He also had no appetite and had lost some weight, but he wasn't sure how much.

"Your answers suggest that you're depressed," Dr. Bergen said, "something that's not unusual after this surgery or any cancer diagnosis. I think we need to do something about this."

"Anything you say, Doc," Lionel said.

Ruby was still in shock after hearing Lionel's responses to the questions. How could she have missed all this? Lionel's agreement to do whatever Dr. Bergen said was also a surprise. He was so passive—in such contrast to his usual feisty self.

Dr. Bergen had turned to the computer on his desk and was busy typing something.

"Honey, Lionel . . . I'm so sorry that I didn't notice how you were feeling . . . I feel terrible!"

Lionel just shook his head. He'd surprised himself when he'd acknowledged how he was feeling in his answers to the doctor's questions. He'd never seen himself as someone who'd get depressed, and when Dr. Bergen had named it, it had come as a shock. Men weren't supposed to get depressed—that was what he'd always believed. His father had fought in the First World War, and even that hadn't affected him, so why was Lionel feeling so bad after a simple operation?

Cancer of the penis and surgery to remove part or all of the penis can have a profound impact on a man's masculinity and body image. This surgery often means the man has to pass urine differently; for example, if the entire penis is removed, he needs to sit to urinate because the urethra will open on the perineum (the space between the scrotum and anus). He may no longer be able to have an erection or penetrative intercourse or even masturbate. But with a partial penectomy, he may still be able to engage in sexual intercourse and have an orgasm.

Dr. Bergen turned back to the couple. "I've prescribed an antidepressant for you, Lionel. You can pick up the pills later this afternoon at the drugstore. It can take two or three and sometimes up to six weeks before you notice any change in your mood. The medication can also have a range of side effects, and the pharmacist will give you a detailed list of those. The list is long, and you likely won't have most of them, so please don't panic. When taking medications for depression or anxiety, it's also helpful to see a therapist, where you can talk about any issues or concerns you might have. I'll leave a list of providers at the front desk for you to take home. Is there anything else we should talk about?"

"No, I think we covered it all, Doc. We've taken up enough of your time." With that, Lionel got up from the chair, wincing a little because the surgical site was still tender.

Ruby wanted to ask more questions, but it was clear that Lionel had had enough, so they left, and she drove them home.

Later that afternoon, Ruby asked Lionel whether he wanted to go with her to pick up the medication Dr. Bergen had prescribed, but he told her he was tired and needed to nap. She wanted him to start taking the pills as soon as possible, so she went alone, even though a little voice in her head told her Lionel really should have talked to the pharmacist himself. He took the first pill that evening before bed; he threw away the paper bag the bottle of pills had come in, along with the document that included instructions for taking the medication and potential side effects and warnings.

After he'd been taking the antidepressant for almost three weeks, Ruby noticed a slight change in her husband. His appetite had improved, and he was less withdrawn; he was still tired a lot of the time, but he had shown some interest in seeing friends again. He had an appointment with Dr. Bergen set for 10 days later, and Ruby told him she'd go with him.

"I'm not a child!" Lionel protested. "You don't have to come with me to every appointment! I can speak for myself after all!"

"I'm coming with you because I need to hear what Dr. Bergen has to say," Ruby said, "not because you need me to!"

What Lionel didn't tell Ruby was that there was something he wanted to talk to his physician about that he didn't want her to know. He thought about how to get some private time with Dr. Bergen, but he couldn't figure out how to make this happen. At the clinic, an opportunity presented itself when the nurse said she needed to weigh him, and she took him to the scale out of earshot of the waiting room.

"Can you ask Dr. Bergen if I can have some time alone with him? There's something private I want to talk about."

"Of course. I'll let him know, and he can figure out how to do that." The nurse was used to this kind of a request, usually from teenagers who wanted to talk about birth control without their accompanying parent knowing.

When Lionel was called into the exam room, Dr. Bergen suggested to Ruby that she spend a few minutes in the waiting room while he examined Lionel. Ruby was a little taken aback, but she turned around and took a seat again.

In the exam room, Dr. Bergen turned to Lionel. "What's bothering you today?"

Lionel cleared his throat. He wasn't sure how to talk about what was bothering him.

Patients are often not asked about any sexual side effects of cancer treatments,[5] and usually they have to raise the topic themselves, despite their discomfort. Research has shown that patients indicate this is an area of unmet need in their treatment.[6]

"So, Doc . . . no one talked to me about this before or after the surgery. But with what's happened, to my . . . you know . . ." He gestured toward his genitals. Dr. Bergen nodded, indicating he understood Lionel wanted to talk about something to do with the surgery. "Well, I tried to . . . you know . . . I tried to . . . um, to see if it still worked . . ." Lionel's face felt hot; this was really difficult to talk about.

"Ah," Dr. Bergen said, "so you tried to see if you could have an erection?"

Lionel nodded, relieved the physician had said the words. "You know, before the surgery, Ruby and I still . . . you know . . . still did it, maybe just once a month or so . . ."

"And you were wondering if you could still have intercourse?" Dr. Bergen seemed to be trying to make the conversation as easy as possible for Lionel, and he was grateful.

"I guess so, Doc," he said. "But see, the problem is that, well, I couldn't you know . . . I didn't . . . finish?"

"You couldn't have an orgasm—in other words, reach a climax?" Dr. Bergen helpfully filled in the words again.

Lionel nodded. He was sure his face was reflecting how difficult this conversation was.

Dr. Bergen took some time explaining to the older man that what he'd experienced was not out of the ordinary. His inability to have an orgasm could be a single event and not something that would continue. It could be a side effect of the surgery, or it could be related to the antidepressant he was taking.

Lionel was confused—why had no one told him about this?

Side effects from medications are common, and that's why you need to be fully informed before you start taking any new medication. In addition to speaking with your doctor, you should also read the written information you get from the pharmacist; many pharmacists also offer individual education when you pick up your prescription. With many antidepressants, sexual side effects are common; these include loss of sexual interest or desire as well as an inability to have an orgasm. Unfortunately, many older people aren't told about this because it's assumed anyone in their 70s or beyond is too old for sex, which is simply not true.

"Can I stop taking the pills?" Lionel asked. "I'm not sure it's worth it if we can't . . ."

"I hear you," Dr. Bergen said, "but I'm worried about your mental health. If you continue to be depressed, that's also going to interfere with your sex life. And your wife really needs to be part of this conversation. I think we should get her back in the room with us."

The physician picked up the phone, pressed one of the buttons, and asked the receptionist to send Ruby to the exam room. When she came in, Dr. Bergen explained what he and Lionel had talked about.

"Oh, for goodness sake!" Ruby looked annoyed that Lionel wanted to stop taking the antidepressant because of the possible impact on their sex life. "I'm done with that, Dr. Bergen! We're not youngsters, obviously, and I'd rather have a husband who is not depressed than have sex!"

Lionel wanted the floor to open up and swallow him. This was so embarrassing, and now he wished he hadn't said anything to Dr. Bergen. Plus, he didn't want their sex life to be over!

"I'm not going to interfere in your relationship," Dr. Bergen said. "This is something the two of you need to sort out, perhaps with a qualified therapist. Lionel, there are also other medications for depression that might not have the same side effects, so it might be time to see a psychiatrist who can better assess what medications might work best for you. In the meantime, there is evidence that regular exercise can be as helpful as medication with mild to moderate depression, and of course exercise has other benefits too. You can try increasing your physical activity as you slowly wean off the medication. But if your depression worsens, you'll need to go back on the pills. You'll also have to be honest about how you're feeling, Lionel. And Ruby, you'll have to watch him closely. How does that sound?"

The American Society of Clinical Oncology (ASCO) publishes guidelines for cancer specialists on a wide variety of symptoms patients might experience, including anxiety and depression. The 2023 guideline[7] on this topic recommends doctors take a stepped approach by suggesting counseling and physical activity to patients as the first interventions. Should these not help, doctors can then prescribe medication.

Ruby was first to answer the doctor. "That sounds like a compromise, Dr. Bergen, and maybe that's the best we can do for now."

But in her mind, this was the start of a serious conversation between her and Lionel, a *private* conversation at that. And it was time to consult mental-health professionals, who would be better versed in how to handle the emotional fallout from Lionel's cancer diagnosis and treatment. While Dr. Bergen had his patient's best interests in mind, he was a family physician, not a specialist in mental health. As a frontline response to Lionel's depression, he was a good starting point, but Ruby thought discussing medications and the emotional trauma Lionel was experiencing was better done with specialists in that field.

KAREN AND DANIEL

Karen, 36, is married to Daniel, and they have two young children. One year ago, she was treated for thyroid cancer; she had surgery to remove the whole thyroid gland, and both the surgeon and medical oncologist told her that, while she would still be monitored carefully, her cancer was effectively cured. There was no evidence of spread to any lymph nodes, or anywhere else in her body, and she didn't need any ongoing treatment, other than taking medication to replace the hormones produced by the thyroid gland.

Initially she was elated with the reassurance from the physicians. Once she recovered from the surgery, she experienced a renewed sense of appreciation for her life and a desire to continue as a stay-at-home mom, rather than return to work as a high school teacher.

"The kids are going to be this little for such a short time," she explained to her sister, Janice, who didn't understand her decision. "Life is much less chaotic, and anyway, Dan is supportive, so that's what I—what we—have decided, and that is that!"

Life *was* less chaotic with Karen at home, and they saved money by not having to send the girls to daycare. She organized their day in 30-minute chunks; her need for organization as a teacher hadn't completely disappeared! There was play time, and story time, when she read to them, and park time, as well as music classes three times a week. Their younger daughter, Amy, was just two years old and still needed an afternoon nap. During that time, Karen gave their older daughter, Amanda, aged four, art supplies to get creative with. And while she was busy doing that, Karen prepared their dinner. Daniel had to admit that he liked this change. He came home, like a 1950s man, to freshly bathed children, a calm wife, and dinner almost ready. He mentioned this to Karen one night, who bristled at the description.

"I am no traditional wife! This is *my* choice and not something imposed by you or society!"

Daniel quickly backtracked. "I meant it as a joke—I'm not a 1950s husband by any means! We're partners in this, in every way."

But that wasn't entirely accurate; he was doing less and less for the girls since Karen had decided not to go back to work. Karen seemed to really enjoy being at home, and she was certainly less stressed than before. She didn't have to spend time marking papers or preparing for the next day's classes. Their sex life was also better—sex was more frequent than during the years when the girls had been babies—despite Karen's cancer. The cancer didn't seem to have had a negative impact on that aspect of their life. They didn't talk about her diagnosis or surgery often, and Daniel thought of it as a small blip in their otherwise unremarkable life together.

But over the next few months, Daniel noticed that Karen had changed. She wasn't the same ebullient woman she'd been after the surgery; her mood was quieter when the children weren't around, and she often seemed distracted. When Daniel asked her whether anything was wrong, she denied it and at times responded in anger.

"Why would anything be wrong? I'm fine, the girls are fine . . . are *you* not fine?"

He knew better than to probe further. Over the years of their marriage, he'd learned to not delve deeper once she'd responded to a question. He tended to approach issues with rationality and consideration—a reason for, or response to, his education as an engineer. But there was something definitely off with Karen, and he wasn't sure what to do about it.

Thyroid cancer is sometimes called a "good" cancer because of the high cure rate—almost 100% for cancers found and treated in the early stages. But for anyone diagnosed with this type of cancer, it's still a cancer diagnosis and not "good" in any way.

A couple of days later, Karen mentioned she needed Daniel to stay home with the girls the following week because she had an appointment for a scan.

"Ah!" he thought to himself, "maybe this is why she's been acting like she has. She's been like this before when she has a scan coming up."

The night before the test, Karen didn't sleep. Daniel felt her tossing and turning for the first hour after she came to bed, and then she got up and went downstairs. He could hear her pacing, and while he wanted to go to her, he thought she'd rebuff him, as she had on previous nights before a scan or an appointment with the medical oncologist. When morning came, she was dressed and preparing breakfast for the girls long before they woke up. Daniel had planned to do that and had even imagined making them fresh orange juice and pancakes that looked like smiley faces. But Karen had already made toast and cut up some fruit for them, so he went back to bed, waiting for stirrings from their bedrooms. He usually appreciated how organized Karen was with the girls, but now he felt as if she were being controlling. Was this part of her dealing with her worry about the scan—or something else?

Worry or anxiety about scans is called "scanxiety" by many survivors, and it's a common experience for anyone who's had cancer. Anxiety levels rise in the days or weeks before the appointment and then decline when normal results come back. This anxiety is normal and may decrease or even disappear as time goes by, but for some, scanxiety persists for a long time and may never go away.

Karen left to have the scan, came home hours later, and acted as if her long absence was typical. To Daniel it clearly wasn't, but when he asked her what took so long, she shrugged and didn't reply.

What she didn't tell him was that she was late because she'd been sitting in her car outside the cancer center, unable to move, her thoughts a blur.

Daniel reached out to hug her, fearing she'd heard something bad that she couldn't talk about, but she bristled and moved away. He was shocked; if there was one thing that had always been good between them, it was their physical connection, in and out of the bedroom. As he tried to make sense of her avoiding his hug, he realized they hadn't made love for weeks . . .

"What's going on?" he asked, his voice louder than he'd intended. "You have to talk to me, Karen. I can't take much more of this!"

"More of what?" was her response.

"Look what just happened! I tried to hug you, and you shuddered, literally shuddered. What have I done? I don't understand what I've done. Did you hear something bad today? Is that it?"

Karen didn't answer; she was staring at her feet. When she looked up, there were tears running down her cheeks. "I'm scared, Dan, really scared . . ."

"Scared of what? Is there something you haven't told me? Did something happen when you had your scan? Have you been feeling sick? What is it?"

"I'm just scared of everything . . . what if the cancer is back?" Her voice was a wail, and she didn't seem to care if the children could hear. "The girls are so young . . . who will take care of them? What if they forget me?"

She was sobbing now, her hands over her face, and Daniel hesitated before he engulfed her in his arms. He wasn't sure what had brought this on; she'd been so happy after the surgery when she'd been told she'd been cured. Why was she worried now? What had happened to cause this response at this point?

The fear of recurrence is something many cancer survivors experience, no matter how positive their prognosis is. It's a form of anxiety that's not necessarily rational but rather an emotional response to the trauma of diagnosis and the need to get through treatment. Some survivors can contain this fear and not allow it to take over, while others experience it as a constant state of vigilance, always monitoring physical sensations and fearing that any new pain, cough, or headache means the cancer is back or has spread. This fear can occur immediately after the end of treatment or months or even years later.

Karen and Daniel held each other for a few minutes, and then she pulled away.

"I hate feeling like this!" She had stopped crying. "I don't know what to do about this, but it's the way I feel, and I can't stop it!"

Daniel was now in crisis-control mode. "We're going to get you some help. When are you seeing someone from the cancer center to hear about the scan results?"

"The nurse said someone will call as soon as the results are in . . . and I can look in the patient portal, but I'm too scared."

"Can I look for you?" Daniel had never looked at anything in her electronic health record.

"Yes, of course you can. That might help . . ."

Later that day, Karen logged into the patient portal, and the results were there. Her scans were normal—there was no evidence the cancer was back. Daniel smiled as he read and reread the words on the screen. Karen's face didn't reveal how she was feeling, but she reached out to touch his shoulder. Daniel could feel her hand shaking slightly.

"Karen, love, we have to find a way to prevent this anxiety from happening every time you have a scan. And it seems to be getting worse with every scan you have." Daniel waited for her response; he was afraid she'd be angry at his suggestion.

"I know, I know . . . it's not easy to be in my head," she said, and she wasn't angry at all. "It feels like I haven't slept in weeks, and I'm so sorry that I've put you through this."

"It's not about me—we need to find you some help." Daniel was always good when there was a problem that needed to be solved. "Is there someone you can talk to at the cancer center?"

Karen wasn't sure, but she remembered she had a booklet that someone, a nurse maybe, had given her when she'd first been diagnosed. She'd put it somewhere, and now she went to look for it. She found it along with other pamphlets in a bag she'd stowed at the back of her closet. The booklet's last page had a list of support services and websites.

One of the contacts was for a cancer support group, and before she lost her nerve, Karen called the number. A man answered the phone and introduced himself simply as Kevin. He told Karen he was a psychologist who facilitated the support group for survivors of thyroid cancer. There was a group meeting later the same week, and he encouraged Karen to attend.

"I'm not sure . . ." She looked at Daniel for confirmation that she should go.

"It's worth a shot, love, and it's unlikely to hurt," he said.

Two days later, Karen drove to the support group meeting, her heart pounding. She almost turned around when she reached the parking lot at the cancer center, but she didn't want to disappoint Daniel. She found her way to the right room and was greeted by a tall man with wire-rimmed glasses and long hair in a ponytail. She almost laughed out loud—he looked very much like the school psychologist at the high school where she'd taught.

"Welcome!" he said. "I'm Kevin, and I facilitate this group. May I ask your name?" As she answered, he gestured for her to follow him toward a circle of empty chairs. In the back corner of the room, a group of people were clustered around a table, all of them women and many about her age.

"We're going to start the meeting in a few minutes," Kevin said, "but before that, can you tell me a little bit about you?" His voice was soft, his smile warm, and Karen found herself telling him why she was here—that her anxiety had just gotten to be too much.

"Ah," he said, "does it help to know that we talk at almost every meeting about the fear and anxiety that I'd say everyone experiences once they've been diagnosed?"

"You do?" Karen was surprised; she'd thought she was the only person who felt this way. Maybe this support group really was what she needed . . .

The purpose of support groups is to do just what the name states—to offer support from others who have gone through the same or similar experiences. A support group specific to a certain cancer can be particularly helpful, as can a group of people of similar age or the same gender. And having a professional facilitator can help to lead a productive discussion, rather than the group being just a way for survivors to express their feelings without suggestions for coping or resolution.

Kevin called to the other women to join the circle, and they did so, even as they kept talking to each other. Kevin introduced Karen, and the women then took turns introducing themselves.

When Kevin asked what they wanted to talk about, a woman who'd introduced herself as Sue raised her hand.

"I'm going out on a limb here because we've never talked about this as long as I've been coming to these meetings ... What about sex? Like, who's having it, and why do I feel like I'm the only person on earth who isn't?"

There was silence for a moment, then four other women put up their hands. Karen wasn't one of them—it was way too early for her to open up to a group of strangers.

"My—our—sex life is nonexistent," one woman said.

"Me too!" said another, and then so did many other women. Even those who hadn't raised their hand nodded their head.

"I know I should've done something about this months ago, but, well, life has gotten in the way, and my partner hasn't seemed to notice, and she hasn't complained. So I just let it slide, I guess," volunteered another woman, and once again other women nodded.

The conversation tapered off at that point, and Kevin stepped in. "I know we haven't talked about this much, but sex, or the lack of it, is a pretty common complaint I hear from patients that I see individually. What do *you* think is the reason for this?"

The women offered their thoughts. Two women said they were just too busy raising their kids and looking after their own parent or parents to even think about sex. One woman asked whether it could have something to do with hormones. Another said she was too tired to have sex, that sex was another chore, and she couldn't find the energy to do one more thing. Karen listened in amazement; it was as if they were speaking for her!

There are many reasons why some people don't want to engage sexually, despite loving their partner. The reasons mentioned in the support group are common for busy women who are often working in or out of the home. The impact of hormone changes as a result of thyroid diseases, including cancer and its treatments, cannot be ignored—although there is little research on this. Most people who've been treated for thyroid cancer will be prescribed thyroid hormone replacement, but this doesn't necessarily "fix" the lack of interest in sex.

"Kevin, what can we do about this? We all seem to be in the same boat," said Sue, the woman who'd first raised the topic.

"I knew you were going to ask that!" he replied. "I'm not a sex therapist, but how about I invite someone who specializes in the topic to come and talk at our next meeting?"

The women all nodded.

"Do you want to include your partners in the session, just for the one night?" Kevin asked, looking around the room. "It's probably a good idea for your partners to hear the same information."

"Uh, no!" was the response from Sue. She seemed to be the unofficial leader of the group, and the others quickly agreed with her.

Karen wasn't sure how she felt about Daniel coming to the group. She wasn't sure she was even going to attend beyond this first meeting. While she knew that sex was important for her relationship, what she really wanted to talk about was her anxiety about the cancer coming back—and no one was mentioning that at all.

The conversation carried on for a while, but Karen didn't participate much. As the meeting wound down and the women went their separate ways, Kevin came up to her and asked what she thought about the experience.

She hesitated before answering, not sure whether he'd be offended if she told him the truth. "Um, it was interesting, but I really wanted to hear more about some other stuff . . ."

"Is there something specific you wanted to talk about?" he asked. "We can always meet separately in my office. I have some openings next week if that works for you."

Karen was relieved to hear that; she didn't want to continue to live the way she had been, with constant worry about her cancer—and she knew it wasn't fair to her family. But maybe she would also attend the next meeting, especially if a professional was going to talk about this sex stuff.

The next day she received an email from Kevin letting the group know that the sex therapist he'd mentioned had agreed to come to their meeting in two weeks. She'd told Daniel about what the support group had talked about, and he'd encouraged her to continue attending the meetings. She still wasn't sure, but he'd looked so hopeful when she'd agreed to go to the first meeting that she didn't want to disappointment him by quitting before she'd given it a real try. She had to admit to herself it was helpful to hear that other women were going through the same things she was.

In the meantime, she made an appointment with Kevin at his office—and it went better than she'd expected. The first thing he told her was that she was not going crazy, that many survivors have a fear of the cancer coming back, and that keeping her fear hidden from family and friends wasn't helpful. He also told her that fear of cancer recurrence was more common in women than men and that childcare responsibilities may contribute to this. He offered to give her some reading material about mindfulness meditation (see appendix 1), and he suggested she include some form of physical exercise in her daily life.

"I don't think I want to take pills," she told Daniel after she'd explained to him what Kevin had told her about some alternatives. "I'm going to read more about mindfulness, and maybe I'll get into yoga too."

Daniel couldn't stop smiling for the rest of the evening, and Karen felt lighter than she had for ages. She hadn't realized how much her anxiety had taken over her life, but now she could see the beginning of something else. "This must be what hope feels like," she thought, "and it feels good."

CONCLUSION

Anxiety and depression are common in those newly diagnosed with cancer, and one or both conditions may persist for months or even years. These are serious mental health issues for anyone but especially so for those with cancer, where they're associated with an increase in death rates.[8]

If you're experiencing anxiety for any reason, it's important to get professional help. Talk therapy such as cognitive behavioral therapy, or CBT, can be very effective in controlling anxiety.

Practicing mindfulness meditation is another helpful strategy (see appendix 1). Exercise, yoga, and music therapy may also help to reduce symptoms. Some people need additional treatment, and there are a variety of prescription medications you can try under the care of a medical professional with expertise in mental health.

TAKEAWAYS

- Depression and anxiety are common after a cancer diagnosis and treatment. There is no timetable for these issues—they can start immediately after your diagnosis, during or after treatment, and even months later.

- Depression and anxiety may coexist; depression may cause anxiety for some people, and feeling anxious may lead to depression. Some medications are designed to treat symptoms of both.

- Anxiety and depression can have significant impacts on daily life, including sexual impacts. Some people avoid sexual activity, while others may use sex to "self-medicate" in order to feel better, even for a brief time.

- Many of the medications used to treat depression or anxiety have sexual side effects, including loss of sexual interest and the inability to have an orgasm. A mental health professional can work with you to find a medication with fewer or more tolerable side effects.

- Alternatives to medication for treating mild-to-moderate depression and anxiety include mindfulness meditation and exercise—and these may be enough to improve how you're feeling.

- Hiding feelings from family and friends increases feelings of isolation and may make the depression or anxiety worse. If you're hesitant to share your feelings, try taking a small step at first, such as talking to one trusted friend or family member, or your family physician or nurse practitioner.

WEBSITES FOR ADDITIONAL INFORMATION

American Cancer Society
https://www.cancer.org/cancer/managing-cancer/side
-effects/emotional-mood-changes.html
https://www.cancer.org/cancer/types/thyroid-cancer
/detection-diagnosis-staging/survival-rates.html

Cleveland Clinic
https://my.clevelandclinic.org/health/diseases/9296
-sexual-problems-and-depression-

Harvard Health
https://www.health.harvard.edu/womens-health/when
-an-ssri-medication-impacts-your-sex-life

Mayo Clinic
https://www.mayoclinic.org/diseases-conditions
/depression/expert-answers/antidepressants/faq
-20058104

Stanford Medicine
https://med.stanford.edu/survivingcancer/coping-with
-cancer/cancer-coping-with-depression.html

CHAPTER 8

"I can't take it anymore!"

When the Partner Leaves

It's often assumed the partner of the person with cancer will act honorably and selflessly, but not all partners are able to cope with the many changes resulting from cancer treatment. The partner may distance themself from the person with cancer, or they may end the relationship. This kind of turn of events can leave the person with cancer feeling devastated, which may precipitate or worsen depression.

DOMINIC AND SYLVIA

Dominic is a 67-year-old widower who, for the past year, has been dating Sylvia, a 60-year-old divorced woman. They met on a dating app for seniors, and after the initial attraction they both felt, they settled in to an easy relationship centered on their mutual love of travel and adventure. They went on a two-week cruise through the Mediterranean, sleeping in separate cabins at first, but within a week, they moved into one of the cabins together. They were a little concerned about what the housekeeping staff would think, but their delight in each other quickly overcame any feelings of shame.

After the cruise, they planned to spend two months in Arizona to escape the winter cold in New Hampshire, where they both lived. They arranged a rental condo, then drove down over four days, and the car trip was filled with laughter and stops at roadside diners, where they ate more burgers and fries than they liked to admit.

Their stay in Arizona was cut short when, three weeks in, Dominic developed a cough that persisted despite two rounds of antibiotics and repeated negative COVID-19 tests. He had a chest X-ray at the urgent care center close to their condo, and the result showed a large lesion in his right lung. They immediately left for the four-day drive back to New Hampshire. There was no laughter this time, and neither of them had any appetite for burgers and fries.

Dominic started treatment for stage 3 lung cancer soon after they got back home. He initially had chemotherapy followed by radiation, and he was told that for now the cancer was under control. Sylvia had moved into his house when he'd started treatment; she'd wanted to take care of him, and he was grateful she'd been there to drive him to his appointments and cook the meals he needed, even though he hardly ate and felt guilty she'd gone to so much trouble to make his favorite dishes.

Most lung cancers (80–85%) are classified as non-small cell lung cancer (NSCLC), and 10–15% are small cell lung cancers (SCLC).[1] *The biggest risk factor is smoking tobacco, but exposure to second-hand smoke or environmental smoke is also a risk. Exposure to radon gas or asbestos is another risk factor, and if you have a family history of lung cancer, your risk of developing the same cancer is higher.*

Treatment for lung cancer depends on the stage and grade of the cancer. It may include surgery to remove the tumor and part or all of the affected lung, radiation, chemotherapy, targeted therapy, or immunotherapy.[2]

Dominic and his wife hadn't been able to have children of their own, and he'd hoped that Sylvia's two children, Lesley and Ethan, would become the family he'd always wanted. Lesley and Ethan were both married with two kids each and had moved to different states after college. They were busy and didn't visit their mother often. Their contact with Sylvia was mostly over the phone, with the occasional FaceTime for birthdays and anniversaries, so their relationship with Dominic was superficial at best.

Sylvia hadn't told Dominic that both Lesley and Ethan had expressed concerns when she'd traveled to Arizona with him. After his cancer diagnosis, they'd suggested to her that she was being "saddled" with a dying man and that the situation wasn't going to bring her much happiness.

Sylvia denied this assessment, but she had started to consider her relationship with Dominic. He'd changed during his treatment—he was tired all the time now—and she hoped this was temporary, but she wasn't sure it would be. She didn't go with him to any of his appointments, other than dropping him off. Instead she waited for him in the parking lot, using the time to read or call a friend. He never said much about what his oncologist told him, so she was unaware of what to expect. She just accepted that he was tired after his radiation treatments and that the chemotherapy sessions made the fatigue worse. She told herself this wasn't forever—he'd recover from the effects of his treatments. But so far he was left with severe shortness of breath and pain on the right side of his chest where the lung cancer had been found.

Depending on your treatment, you can experience different side effects. These include fatigue from radiation or chemotherapy, throat and mouth sores from chemotherapy, skin reactions from im-muno- or targeted therapy, shortness of breath, cough, hair loss, diarrhea, or constipation. The oncology care team should pro-vide you with information about possible side effects and how to manage them.

At the end of the summer, Sylvia asked Dominic where he wanted to spend the upcoming winter. She was shocked at his response.

"I don't think I want to go anywhere this winter," he said, seemingly unaware this might upset her. "I'm so damn tired, and the thought of driving all the way—"

"We don't have to drive," she interrupted. "We can fly to Phoenix and rent a car."

"But that's not the only thing," he said. "How am I going to get travel insurance now?"

She hadn't thought about that, but she wasn't going to give up so easily. "You can still buy insurance! It might cost a bit more but—"

"But nothing! It'll cost a bomb, and anyway, I'm not sure my doctor will clear me to go away for that length of time."

Sylvia had run out of counterarguments. She was frustrated with him, and she was not looking forward to the long, cold winter in New Hampshire. Later, on the phone with her daughter, Sylvia mentioned that she and Dominic weren't going to Arizona this year.

"Why not?" Lesley said. "I thought you hated winter and one of the reasons you retired was so you could go away for the worst of it!" Lesley's tone was a bit harsh.

But as they talked, Sylvia's frustration grew. The reality was she didn't want to spend the winter here in the cold and snow, but she also didn't know what to do about the situation. When she and Dominic had met, she'd been so happy to find someone interested in the same things she was. Sure, he was 67 years old, but he was young at heart and a good match energy-wise for her at 60. But the cancer had aged him, and the 7-year difference between them now seemed much bigger.

Aging is the most important risk factor for the development of cancer, and cancer plays a role in the aging process.[3] *Most cancers develop after age 50 as damage naturally occurs to cells in the body. In addition, immunity decreases as we age, and our body is less efficient in detecting and fighting cancer cells. People with cancer also experience frailty and chronic diseases at a younger age than those without cancer; this is evidence of their accelerated aging.*

Sylvia thought about finding an alternative to going to Arizona and made a couple of suggestions to Dominic, but he rejected every one of them. He continued to cough, and although his oncologist had ordered home oxygen for him, the machine sat in the corner of the dining room gathering dust. He didn't complain, but she could see he was in pain because he winced when he moved, even though he tried to hide it from her. She was still living with him, but they no longer shared a bed. Dominic preferred to sleep sitting in a recliner that he'd bought when he'd found that lying flat increased his shortness of breath.

It didn't help that both Lesley and Ethan had raised the topic of Sylvia getting out of the relationship or at least returning to her own condo, which she'd rented out on a month-by-month basis. She'd responded with a firm no to their suggestion, but it had planted a seed . . .

A call from her sister in Los Angeles prompted Sylvia to come up with a compromise. She would go for a two-week visit to see her sister in the new year, giving herself a break from the New Hampshire winter. Dominic seemed fine with the plan, and Sylvia was more relieved than she'd expected to be. Lesley and Ethan also sounded happy when she told them, and she hoped this new plan would stop them from nagging her about not traveling very much.

She flew to Los Angeles, her anticipation growing when she thought about the warmer days and relaxing with her sister, who had a lovely home and a housekeeper who was a great cook. These thoughts were tempered by her feelings of guilt over leaving Dominic. But he'd assured her that he would be fine. He'd promised to call her every day and had insisted he'd manage fine with the meals she'd prepared and put in the freezer.

The first week was as good as Sylvia had hoped; the weather was beautiful, and she and her sister went on long walks in the morning around the neighborhood, then frequently went out for lunch. They made plans to spend a night or two in Santa Barbara at the same hotel they'd stayed in years before to celebrate Sylvia's divorce.

Dominic called each day as he'd promised, but he sounded awful. He was coughing a lot, and he was also wheezing, a new symptom that had developed since she'd left. He tried to hide it, but she could hear he was struggling to breathe. She made the decision to leave California and return home to be with him. Her sister was upset, and Lesley was clearly frustrated with her choice.

"Why do you always put others before yourself, Mother?" Lesley's use of the word "mother" reflected how angry her daughter was.

"Lesley, I'm not a child! I cannot in good conscience stay here when Dominic needs me."

This did not help.

"Why does he need you?" Lesley said. "It's not like you have a committed relationship!"

"You know nothing about our relationship and how committed it is or isn't! I'm leaving this afternoon, and that's all there is to it!"

Sylvia ended the call and immediately began to cry. Lesley's words weren't completely off base. Sylvia had been thinking about how things had changed with Dominic, and she found herself wondering what she had gotten herself into. There had been no "in sickness and in health" clause when they'd talked about their future a year ago!

Family members and friends often become informal caregivers, and they can carry a range of burdens in the caregiver role. According to the National Alliance for Caregiving (NAC), at least 53 million Americans are providing care for someone with cancer. The impacts of this kind of caregiving include depression, sleep deprivation, social isolation, loss of identity, financial burden, and multiple changes to usual life.[4]

The flight back to New Hampshire through New York was not easy. Sylvia alternated between feeling guilty about leaving Dominic alone for the visit with her sister and wanting relief from the caregiving responsibilities she knew awaited her. Things had looked so different one year ago when they'd met . . .

As she'd feared, Dominic wasn't in good shape when she finally dragged her suitcase into his condo. She was bone tired, both physically and emotionally, and he looked awful. His lips were tinged with blue at the corners, and he was struggling to breathe. He hadn't called his medical providers, and it looked as if he hadn't moved off the recliner for days. She had been gone for just a week, and in that time his condition had deteriorated significantly.

Despite his protests, she called the number for the cancer center where he'd been treated. They told her to take him to the emergency department—and to call an ambulance if she couldn't get him into her car. He refused to leave the condo, and she wasn't sure he could make it to the elevator, then the parking garage and her car, so she called 911. The paramedics arrived within 10 minutes, started him on oxygen, and lifted him onto a stretcher and out the doors to the waiting ambulance. By now it was close to midnight, and she was too exhausted to follow them, so she lay down on the sofa and was asleep in minutes.

Early the next morning she awoke to the sound of her phone ringing. It was her son, Ethan, and he had a lot to say. "This isn't what you signed up for, Mom! Lesley called me last night to tell me that you'd cut short your time in Los Angeles, and frankly, I don't really understand why you did that."

Sylvia was barely awake, and she let him continue as she tried to pull her response together.

"This is nuts, what you've gotten yourself into. You're a nursemaid after a few months with him, and all your own plans have gone by the wayside. Get out now, cut your losses, and put yourself first for a change! You can come and stay with us, or stay with Lesley and her family until your renter leaves. But you need to get out of this situation!" Sylvia didn't argue with him—she was still too exhausted. But she told him she'd think about what he'd said, then she hung up.

Sylvia showered and dressed, then drove to the hospital, his words repeating in her mind. A nurse from the emergency department had left a message for her in the early hours of the morning; Dominic was being admitted to the palliative care unit to control his symptoms. Sylvia wasn't sure what this meant. Would he be able to go home at some point, and what did that mean for her? She wasn't convinced she'd be able to leave their relationship, but she also didn't want to be tied down because of guilt. She sat in the car outside the hospital as she wrestled with her feelings. No matter what she decided, she was going to feel bad. Staying with Dominic had caused a rift with her daughter and son—the last thing she wanted. Ethan was correct in that her relationship with Dominic was relatively new, and caring for a sick and dying man was not what Sylvia had signed up for. But if she left him, she'd feel terribly guilty. He had no one other than her to help him, and she wasn't sure how long he'd stay in hospital. She had no one to talk to about her feelings; her children had obviously determined she should leave Dominic. But what she needed was someone who could be objective, who could listen to her and support her in whatever decision she made. In that moment a potential answer came to her; she would talk to someone who worked in the unit where Dominic was admitted and ask them whether there was a professional who could help her. She had a plan, or the beginning of a plan, and she opened the car door with the sense that she was doing something to help herself in a difficult situation—at least she hoped so.

BECKA AND DEVON

Becka was the 34-year-old partner of Devon, who had an aggressive brain tumor. Since starting treatment, he'd been acting out of character, and at times he was verbally abusive to her.

Not only was she concerned the abuse would become physical, but she also found she didn't want to have sex with him anymore—he seemed like a stranger to her now, not the man she'd married.

Before his diagnosis, Becka and Devon had been married for 10 years. They had two children, 8-year-old Jack and 5-year-old Adele. Together they owned a flower shop; Becka was responsible for ordering the flowers and creating arrangements, and Devon managed the accounts and their website. Becka noticed something was wrong when Devon started forgetting to invoice their business customers. One of their longtime clients called the store and told Becka that it had been two months since they'd been asked for payment for the weekly floral arrangements they received. Becka checked the bank statements and found that Devon hadn't invoiced any of their clients for the previous couple of months. When she asked him about it, he denied he hadn't sent out invoices.

There were other signs too. Devon started to have headaches that lasted two to three days. Then he forgot to pick up the kids from his parents' place after a sleepover. Becka had to deliver flowers for a wedding that morning, and she was irritated when his mother called her to say the kids were still at her house and she needed to go to her weekly bridge game. When Becka texted Devon to remind him that he needed to get the kids from his mother, he accused her of not telling him that they'd slept over there. This was really strange—didn't he realize the children hadn't slept at home the night before?

She and Devon had also started arguing more, mostly about little things that previously hadn't caused conflict. As the weeks went by, the arguments grew more and more frequent, and Devon had started to say really mean things to her. It was summer, and this was their busy season with weddings almost every weekend. Driving to and from wedding venues, Becka thought about the signs that something might be really wrong with Devon. Finally, after an intense argument with him over something trivial—he had neglected to buy cat food for the third time—she insisted that he see their family physician. Despite his protests that there was nothing wrong with him and that she was making things up, she made an appointment for him with Dr. Simon.

There are different kinds of malignant brain tumors, including astrocytoma, glioblastoma (the most common malignant brain tumor), ependymoma, and oligodendroglioma. Primary brain tumors are those that start in the brain; other cancers can spread to the brain and are then called "metastases" of the original cancer.

Symptoms of brain cancer depend on the size of the tumor, where it's located, and how fast it's growing. Symptoms may include headaches or pressure in the head that's worse in the morning; nausea and vomiting; blurry or double vision; balance problems; or symptoms related to brain function, such as confusion or memory loss, personality or behavior changes, and seizures.

In general, the risk of developing a brain tumor is 1%.[5]

Devon never made it to his appointment. Three days before he was due to see Dr. Simon, Becka came home from a delivery to find him unconscious on their en suite bathroom floor. He had blood on his face from biting his tongue, and he had wet himself. The children were at the park with their babysitter and had fortunately not witnessed this. Becka called 911, her hands shaking and her voice high pitched and panicked. The paramedics were there within minutes, and she went with Devon to the hospital. There, a CT scan showed a tumor in his brain the size of a lime.

Within days he saw a number of cancer specialists, and a treatment plan was made.

First there was radiation and chemotherapy to shrink the tumor, and then he had surgery. Through all this, Becka had to support their children, who were shell-shocked by what was happening to their father. She also had to try and keep herself calm, while running the store and filling orders. She was exhausted, barely eating, and on the verge of panic most of the time.

Devon's treatment regimen was challenging, to say the least. He barely slept owing to the large doses of steroids he was taking to counteract the effects of the radiation and chemotherapy. And it wasn't as if he stayed in bed when he was awake during the night. He got up and wanted to go outside, and she was scared he would hurt himself. He was unsteady on his feet and had fallen a couple of times, fortunately not hitting his head, but he'd gotten a series of bumps and bruises on his limbs.

The worst part was his anger, which hadn't gone away as the tumor shrank—in fact, his anger had grown. The doctor had warned her this could happen, and it was common in patients with brain cancer. He flew into rages at the slightest provocation; a request from Becka to put his empty mug in the sink or Jack asking him to play outside led to him screaming at them. The children knew something was wrong with their dad, but they didn't fully understand the seriousness of his condition. When he yelled at Becka, they ran to their bedrooms or the backyard, their faces showing their confusion and terror at the storm of his anger. He'd started calling Becka names and accusing her of ruining their business. One night he called her a "nasty bitch" during dinner, and when she told him that wasn't appropriate, he pushed her against the dining-room wall, his right arm across her throat. The children saw the whole thing and tried to pull him away from her. Their pleas for him to leave their mother alone finally got through, and he let her go. She slumped against the wall, tears streaming down her face, her arms reaching out to shelter the children from him.

This was the last straw. The next day Becka called the social worker assigned to him at the cancer center.

The social worker, Elizabeth, had met Becka and Devon once when he'd been newly diagnosed. She'd given them her contact information with an open invitation for either of them to request support at any time. She wasn't surprised to hear from Becka; it was common for couples coping with brain cancer to experience challenges.

Family caregivers experience a range of challenges when caring for their loved one, and it's often more stressful for the caregiver than the person with cancer. The personality and behavior changes are particularly difficult to cope with. Family caregivers experience high rates of anxiety and depression, loneliness, difficulty adjusting to the changes, and poor quality of life.[6]

Two days later, Becka met with Elizabeth, who noted Becka seemed tense and exhausted.

"Tell me what's going on at home," the social worker said as soon as they sat down.

"I . . . I . . . don't know where to start." Becka's voice was shaky. "It's like he's a different person. His anger is like a tornado . . . he goes from 0 to 120 in seconds, and it terrifies the kids."

Elizabeth nodded as Becka spoke. She'd heard similar stories from the partners of people with brain cancer multiple times over the years. "Has there been physical violence along with the anger?" she asked gently.

Becka looked at the social worker with terror in her eyes. How did the social worker know? She nodded and tried to find the words to describe how scared she'd been when Devon had pushed her against the wall. "The other day . . . he pushed me against the wall . . . it was terrifying."

"Can you tell me more about what happened?" Elizabeth had a feeling there was more to what Becka had gone through than what she'd managed to say so far.

Becka was silent. She'd already replayed the incident over and over in her head, and putting it into words now brought back the physical sensations. "I don't know what started it. I might have said something . . . Oh yes, he had called me a bitch or something, and I called him out. The next thing I knew, he had me against the wall, and it felt like I was going to pass out . . . the kids were screaming, and that's all I remember."

"So, your children saw this?" Elizabeth's tone reflected her concern. It was one thing for Devon to put his hands on his wife, but for the children to witness this elevated the direness of what had happened.

Becka nodded; now she was sobbing, her hands over her face.

"Has there been anything else?"

Becka nodded again. She knew she had to tell the social worker everything that had been going on, but what she had to disclose was hard to put into words. "He wants to have sex all the time . . . and he doesn't seem to care when and where he wants it. He grabs me if I get close enough for him to touch me . . . and he does this in front of the kids too."

"He grabs you? Can you explain what you just said?" Elizabeth wasn't being nosey; she needed to know the details to assess the situation fully.

"He grabs my breasts all the time . . . and my butt . . . and this is not like him. At least, it's not like he used to be . . . he was always so gentle and respectful." Once she'd started talking, Becka couldn't stop. "He's my husband and I love him, but I can't have sex with him—not like he is now! It's like he's someone else."

Tumors in the frontal lobe of the brain are often associated with behavior and personality changes such as loss of inhibitions, which result in inappropriate behavior.[7] "Sexual disinhibition" refers to the lowering of the usual "brakes" on sexual behavior. The person may behave in an inappropriate manner, such as demanding sex from a partner, masturbating in front of others, or touching others in a sexual way. This has a negative impact on the family, especially on the partner, who may feel overwhelmed and isolated as other supports wane because of people's reluctance to deal with the patient's behavior. The behavior may decrease or disappear after the treatment phase is over and the tumor has been removed or has shrunk considerably.

Elizabeth took a deep breath. She knew what she was going to suggest to Becka wasn't going to be easy for the woman to hear. "Becka, I'm concerned for your safety and the safety of your children." She waited a moment before continuing. She wanted Becka to have heard what she said and to be prepared for what she was going to say next. "What is happening in your home and with your husband is common when someone has brain cancer. It's like they become someone else, and it may get worse, at least in the short term."

Becka was staring at the social worker as she spoke. Hearing the words was a wake-up call for her but also confirmation of what she already knew. The situation at home was indeed dangerous for her and for their children. The thought of Devon hurting the children in any way was horrifying, and as much as she had pushed that thought away, the social worker was right.

"I encourage you to get out of this situation immediately," Elizabeth said. "Is there somewhere you and the kids can go?"

Becka couldn't answer. She was overwhelmed and couldn't think straight.

Elizabeth continued. "It may only be for a couple of days or weeks . . ."

"But how can I leave him?" Becka said. "He needs me. Who's going to look after him? What if he falls or has another seizure? What then?" Her voice was a wail.

Elizabeth took Becka's hands and held them tight. "The team here who's treating him—we'll help you figure it out. But you and the kids need to be safe. Do you understand that? I'm worried for all three of you. And for your husband, of course. But you're not going to be able to help him if you are harmed."

That last sentence got through to Becka, and she felt a sense of calm, like a cool wave, settle over her body. "The kids can go to my mother-in-law. She's good in a crisis, and the kids love her, and she adores them. I can stay with a friend for a few days. But how can Devon be at home alone?"

"I'm going to talk to his doctor. We'll see if we can get him admitted to hospital for a full psychiatric assessment, and hopefully some new medication or an adjustment to what he's on now. That way you and the kids can return home while he's in hospital, but the plan all depends on what the medical team can do."

"You can make that happen?" Becka felt some hope from Elizabeth's response. But she also felt guilty that things had come to this. She loved Devon deeply and was so sad he needed to be in hospital, but she also knew that she and the kids, and Devon too, needed to be safe.

"I will try my hardest," Elizabeth said. "As I said before, this isn't the first time I've dealt with this kind of situation, and the medical team has always been helpful. If you're agreeable, let me make a few phone calls while you wait with a cup of coffee or tea—it shouldn't take long."

Up to 20% of patients with brain tumors need admission to a hospital for in-patient care, and of those, 37% will die within six months.[8] Caring for someone with a brain tumor is extremely demanding for family caregivers, many of whom feel unprepared to provide the level of care that's needed.[9]

Before she'd met with Elizabeth, Becka had taken the children to their grandmother's, and now, while she was waiting for Elizabeth to return, she needed to check on them. Her mother-in-law's tone when she answered the phone told Becka that the kids—or more likely, Adele, the five-year-old—had told their grandmother what Devon had done the night before.

"Becka, honey, are you okay? This is just awful!" her mother-in-law said. "I don't know what to say, but I think the kids need to stay with me for a few days—until this gets sorted out. I am so, so sorry this is happening to you! I had no idea . . ."

As Becka had told Elizabeth, her mother-in-law was great in a crisis, and this was certainly a crisis, and it had been for a while. But Becka had tried to minimize or deny the difficulties she'd been dealing with.

Elizabeth came back into the room, so Becka thanked her mother-in-law and ended the call.

"I talked to your husband's doctor," Elizabeth said, "and he agrees with me that we need to get Devon into hospital for an assessment. There's a bed available now, and we need to act quickly. The physician assistant—I think his name is Jose—who works with the oncologist is going to call Devon and ask him to come in to see the team. Do you feel safe going home and driving him to the cancer center?" Elizabeth was concerned about this part of the plan, but there was no other way of getting Devon to see the oncologist and be admitted.

"I think it'll be okay," Becka replied. "It's not like he's angry all the time. And he's told me that he really likes Jose, so hopefully he'll agree to go in and see them. And I just spoke to my mother-in-law, and she's of course more than willing to have the kids for a few days . . . but if he's admitted to hospital, the kids and I can stay at home, right?"

"Yes, that's right," Elizabeth said. She knew this was a stop-gap solution, and she hoped that, with the right medication, Devon could return home to his family.

Unfortunately, Devon's condition did not improve. He had a CT scan soon after he was admitted to hospital that showed the tumor had grown despite treatment. His behavior didn't improve, and the psychiatrist that assessed him concluded he posed a danger to his family and himself. Becka was faced with the reality that she and the children could no longer live with Devon. This felt as though she were abandoning him, and the guilt was overwhelming. She visited him every day in the hospital, and at first he begged her to take him home. She tried to explain to him that he couldn't come home, but one day this made him so angry the staff needed to intervene. She cried as she drove home, the feelings of guilt so all-encompassing that she almost turned back to get him released. His begging to go home and her overwhelming guilt in response went on for two weeks; she wasn't sleeping, and she struggled to keep up with the orders for floral arrangements from their business clients. She'd reluctantly closed the flower shop to casual customers, but she was still barely managing to cope.

It's common for family caregivers of people with a brain tumor to struggle with many aspects of living with their loved one.[10] They experience anxiety and uncertainty about the future and the changed nature of the relationship, and they face challenges finding social support for themselves and putting the needs of the patient ahead of their own.

And then there were the children. They had visited their father in hospital once when he was first admitted, but it had been traumatic for them. Jack, the eight-year-old, had refused to go back after that one visit, when Devon hadn't recognized him. Adele, at five years old, had just been confused about why her father wasn't at home. Both children had been in tears in the car on the way home, and Becka had decided that no one had benefited from their visit. This made her feel even more guilty, but her mother-in-law once again came to the rescue and told Becka that the children didn't need to see their father in that condition. Becka ached for the older woman who, despite what had happened to her only son, put the children first.

Devon's condition continued to deteriorate. He started having seizures three then five times a day, and the medication to control the seizures was so sedating that he slept most of the time. It was rare for Becka to find him awake when she visited him; the social worker and nursing staff encouraged her to take some time for herself and limit her visits to just once or twice a week. Becka knew they were right; she was exhausted all the time, but she was also torn, and the guilt ate at her. The safety instructions on every plane ride she'd taken came back to her: in order to help her children, she needed to put on her own oxygen mask first. By listening to the advice to take time for herself, she was caring for her children—and herself. She wasn't abandoning Devon, so why did she feel as if she were?

CONCLUSIONS

Caring for someone with cancer places significant burdens on their family caregivers. While most family caregivers act with courage and determination to do everything they can, emotionally and practically, the caregiving burden may exceed their ability to do so. Without additional support, whether informal or professional, doing this alone can be isolating and, above all, exhausting. Well-meaning friends and family may try to persuade the family caregiver to walk away in order to "save" themselves, but this isn't easy to do. Guilt and shame about the decision to stay and care for the person or to leave the situation are common responses to an experience where there are no clear-cut solutions.

TAKEAWAYS

- Caring for someone with advanced cancer places a significant burden on family caregivers.
- Transitions in the care needs of a loved one with cancer can be difficult to deal with.
- Professionals such as social workers are a good resource when someone is struggling with the demands of caring for a loved one with a brain tumor.
- Guilt and shame are common when caregivers need to distance themselves from the demanding responsibilities of care.

WEBSITES FOR ADDITIONAL INFORMATION

American Cancer Society (lung cancer and brain and spinal cord tumors)
https://www.cancer.org/cancer/types/lung-cancer/about/what-is.html
https://www.cancer.org/cancer/types/brain-spinal-cord-tumors-adults/about/key-statistics.html

American Lung Association (lung cancer)
https://www.lung.org/lung-health-diseases/lung-disease-lookup/lung-cancer

Mayo Clinic (lung cancer and brain tumor)
https://www.mayoclinic.org/diseases-conditions/lung-cancer/symptoms-causes/syc-20374620
https://www.mayoclinic.org/diseases-conditions/brain-tumor/symptoms-causes/syc-20350084

National Alliance for Caregiving (NAC)
https://www.caregiving.org

National Cancer Institute (NIH) (lung cancer and brain tumor)
https://www.cancer.gov/types/lung
https://www.cancer.gov/types/brain

CHAPTER 9

"I've been affected too!"

The Impact on the Partner

The impact of cancer on the partner is often not recognized fully; their life, hopes, and dreams can feel shattered by the diagnosis. Witnessing the suffering of a loved one is challenging, but partners are often afraid to voice their own suffering in case they're seen as selfish. Talking about the changes in a couple's sexual relationship remains a taboo for many, and this chapter highlights the impact of these sexual changes on the partner of the person with cancer and the difficulty some of them experience.

ROB AND ANGELA

Rob's wife Angela had a double mastectomy one year ago, and since then they haven't had anything resembling what their sex life was like before. For the first two months after surgery, Rob didn't initiate sex; he understood Angela had been through a lot, and she showed no interest. The aftermath of the surgery was difficult. Angela came home with thick bandages on her chest as well as two drains to collect blood and fluid from the surgical sites. He had to help her bathe and use the toilet, and he did all the cooking and cleaning while she slowly got back to her usual level of functioning.

Within a couple of weeks, the drains were removed and the heavy bandages replaced with smaller and lighter ones. Eventually Angela was left with a flat chest and visible scars. She'd declined reconstruction and instead wanted to "go flat." She'd told Rob of her decision, and while he'd been surprised, he hadn't said anything—it was her body, and she could do what she wanted. He didn't fully understand her choice, but he respected that it was her decision to make. She'd always had small breasts, and he'd loved them even as they'd changed over the years. They became smaller after she'd breastfed their three children, and she'd told him she liked the fact that she could go without a bra most of the time. Angela was one of those women who lost weight as she grew older, and as she'd entered her 60s, she'd become lean, and her Pilates practice had increased her muscles so that she looked like an athlete—and he loved that too.

For weeks after the surgery, Rob didn't even hug her, fearing he'd cause her pain, and she gave no indication she missed any form of physical contact. They'd always been physically affectionate with one another. Angela would tell her friends Rob was like a golden retriever puppy, always ready for a tummy rub or cuddle, and that it was one of the things she loved about him. He in turn appreciated that she never turned him down for sex and sometimes initiated as well. He didn't disclose this to his friends because they were always complaining that their sex lives had been over since their wives had gone through menopause. But things were different now after the surgery, and Rob had no idea when or if they'd go back to the way they'd been before. Most of all, he missed touching Angela and being touched by her.

Touch is essential for both physical and mental well-being, and it leads to feelings of comfort, calm, or pleasure.[1] People who don't experience physical touch describe feeling a "skin hunger." The COVID-19 pandemic, when physical touch was restricted, highlighted the negative impacts of the lack of physical touch.[2] But simple physical touch has also been associated with a decrease in pain, anxiety, and depression.[3]

Angela was told she needed anti-estrogen treatment after the mastectomy, but nothing more, and within three months she seemed almost back to her old self. She returned to the Pilates studio with a vengeance; she complained to Rob that the time away from her practice had her feeling weak and still not herself. She was frustrated that getting back to where she'd been before the surgery was taking so long. Rob tried to empathize, but he found her focus on her physical recovery to be a little obsessive. But he couldn't tell her that. And they still hadn't talked about their lack of physical contact, and he was getting increasingly frustrated, both sexually and emotionally. One morning he decided he'd address his feelings with her.

She came back from her Pilates session with a big smile on her face. "I think I'm finally back to where I was!" she announced as she emptied her water bottle in the sink. "It feels so good, and Tammy is pleased with my progress!" Tammy was her Pilates instructor.

Rob took a deep breath. "Angie, honey, there's something we need to talk about . . ."

Angela had moved to the refrigerator and was filling a glass with ice water. She didn't turn toward him.

"Ange, can you please sit down and at least look at me?" His voice had a whiny tone, so he cleared his throat and tried again. "Angela, I'm talking to you. Please, sit down. There's something we need to discuss!"

At the change in tone, Angela paid attention and sat down across from him. "Okay, what's so important? I need to shower . . ."

Rob had been preparing what he wanted to say in his head, but in the moment now, the words disappeared.

"Seriously, Rob, I need to shower." Angela sounded irritated.

"Okay," Rob started, "it's just that, well, things haven't been the same between us for a while . . ."

Angela didn't say anything. She just looked at him, her eyes narrowed.

Rob found her lack of response uncomfortable, so he kept talking. "We haven't touched since your surgery. Haven't you noticed that? I miss you . . . I miss the way things were . . ."

To his surprise, Angela had tears in her eyes. She wasn't someone who cried easily, so this was unexpected. Rob wasn't sure what to do. She still didn't say anything. She just sat across from him with a look on her face that he hadn't seen before in the 40-plus years of their relationship.

"Ange, honey . . . what is it?" As he said the words, he got up from his chair and reached for her. She didn't stand up, so he stood behind her and put his arms around her shoulders, being careful to avoid her chest. He wasn't sure where he could touch her, so he bent forward awkwardly. Other than when he'd helped her bathing, this was the first time he'd touched her since the surgery. This realization felt like a punch to his chest. He felt himself tearing up as he held her, and he tried to blink the tears away. The two of them stayed in that slightly awkward hug for a few minutes, until Angela started to get up.

"I know, I know," she said, her face showing what her words could not.

To Rob, she looked so sad, and he reached out again to comfort her. Or was he comforting himself?

It's common for the partner of a cancer survivor to have a need for comfort that's equally important as the survivor's supportive care needs. "Emotional support" refers to giving love, reassurance, compassion, and acceptance to a loved one. It's common for the partner to minimize their need for this kind of support in the face of the survivor's distress or needs.

After her shower, Rob tried to talk to Angela again. It wasn't easy for him; he was a man who preferred actions to words, and he was afraid that, if his words weren't clear, her feelings would be hurt. That was the last thing he wanted.

"Honey, I don't want to pressure you," he said, "but it's been ages since we made love . . . and I—"

"Is that all you can think of?"

Rob was startled. Angela's response was even more surprising than her tears earlier. Hadn't he shown her by his actions over the past months that he was focused on her? She sounded so angry now, and he hadn't expected this. He wasn't sure what he had expected—but it hadn't been anger!

He tried again. "Honey, it's just that we hardly ever touch, and we're living like roommates, and I don't want to . . . I can't . . . I can't live like this!" His voice reflected his anguish, and even though he knew his tone would probably result in Angela crying—or worse, getting even more angry—he was desperate at this point. The words seemed to get through to her, and as he'd feared, she started to cry again.

"I miss you too," she managed to say between sobs. "I don't know what's going on, but I've just lost any interest in sex . . . I don't understand why this is happening to me! No one told me it was going to be like this. Why did no one tell me?"

Rob couldn't answer her question. He wasn't sure whether it would matter if he did anyway. He thought back to Angela's cancer diagnosis. It had come as a shock after a routine mammogram had shown a possible lesion in her breast, and a biopsy days later had confirmed she did indeed have breast cancer. They'd both wanted to get the cancer out, as soon as possible, and within 10 days she'd had the operation.

Rob couldn't recall anyone, including the surgeon or a nurse, telling them that after her mastectomy their sex life would cease to exist. "Have you talked to Dr. Robin about this?" he asked.

Dr. Robin was their family physician. They'd started seeing her just before Angela's diagnosis, and Rob had only met the young physician once for an initial "get to know you" appointment. Angela had seen her after her final meeting with the surgeon who'd performed the mastectomy. At that appointment, Dr. Robin had prescribed the anti-estrogen medication Angela would need to take for 10 years. Rob hadn't gone to the appointment; Angela had told him it was no big deal, and she went alone. She hadn't said much after the appointment, so Rob had assumed all was well. But now his experience suggested all was not well, at least in terms of their relationship.

The American Society of Clinical Oncology recommends that women with breast cancer who are postmenopausal and whose breast cancer is hormone- (estrogen-) sensitive receive anti-estrogen therapy for up to 10 years.[4] Estrogen production is blocked to reduce the risk of the cancer recurring. As with most medications, there are side effects, and women who take this medication experience menopausal symptoms, including sexual effects such as vulvar and vaginal dryness as well as loss of interest in sex.

Angela hadn't talked to Dr. Robin about sex after surgery. She admitted to Rob that she was embarrassed to talk about such a private issue. And until he'd raised the topic, she'd been unaware the lack of sex had been affecting him so badly.

Rob was stunned. How could she not know? As he thought about this, he decided he would talk to Dr. Robin on his own, since Angela was too embarrassed. He knew he ran the risk of offending her by leaving her out of the conversation, but he was desperate. A little later, he called the physician's office while he was out on a walk, and he made an appointment for the following week when Angela was at her Pilates class.

Dr. Robin's clinic was a short walk from their house, and the next week, as soon as Angela backed the car out of the driveway for her class, Rob headed out. The clinic had just opened when he arrived, and he was the first patient.

He waited in her office for a few minutes, and then Dr. Robin entered.

"Rob, hello!" she said. "Is it okay to call you by your first name?"

"Sure thing, Dr. Robin. It's nice to see you, but I'm not here for myself . . . no, that's not quite right . . . this is about me . . . but really about me and Angela . . . and oh, I'm babbling."

Dr. Robin smiled as she sat down in her chair across from Rob, whose face was now looking quite flushed. She had a feeling this appointment was going to be longer than the 15 minutes allotted. "So, tell me what's going on with you and Angela."

Rob told her about Angela's surgery and recovery, and the physician waited patiently. He knew it was taking him a while to get to the crux of the matter.

After a few minutes, Dr. Robin gently interrupted him. "How has all of this affected *you*, Rob?"

That simple question came as a surprise to him; all these months, his focus had been almost entirely on Angela, until the lack of sex had become unbearable to him. "I don't really know how to answer that. It wasn't me with the cancer!"

"But cancer isn't just an individual experience—it affects both of you," Dr. Robin said. She could tell there was something in particular this man wanted to talk about, but he was struggling to get the words out. "You don't have to feel guilty about what you feel, Rob. This is your experience too, although obviously in a different way."

This was the invitation Rob needed. He told her that since her surgery, Angela hadn't been interested in sex, or seemingly in any physical contact at all, and that he was confused and bothered and sad about this. He told her that their sex life had been so good before the cancer. "It may seem unusual to you," he said, "an older couple who still enjoyed an active sex life, but we did, and it was great. And now . . . nothing!" He explained that neither he nor Angela was happy about this, but they didn't know what to do.

Among older adults, 20 to 30% continue to be sexual, even into their 80s.[5] The most common reason for older adults to not be sexually active is due to their health or the health of their partner. The most common reason for older women not being sexually active is the absence of a partner.

"I'm glad to hear that, Rob," Dr. Robin said. "There's no reason why two healthy adults in their 60s shouldn't enjoy sex. But as you've discovered, cancer and its treatments can change that, and you've done the right thing by asking for help. At least, I think that you're asking . . ."

Rob nodded. He was relieved the topic was out in the open, and he hoped Dr. Robin could offer him some advice.

"This is something that ideally we'd talk about with Angela here. Do you think she'd be willing for the two of you to come and see me? I can certainly answer any questions you have today, but solutions will only happen if both of you are on the same page."

"I think she'll come to see you," Rob said, "and hopefully with me, but in the meantime, can you give me an idea about what's causing her to be disinterested?"

"There are many different reasons why Angela may be experiencing a lack of interest. A diagnosis of cancer is a life-changing event. The surgery she had, the double mastectomy, is itself a big deal, both physically and emotionally. For a woman, her breasts are part of her sexuality and sense of femininity. And of course, Angela is taking the anti-estrogen medication, which has physical and sexual side effects."

"Yeah, that's something we talked about," Rob said. "But she never told me much about the medication other than that she'd need to take the pills for 10 or so years."

Dr. Robin tried to hide a sigh. She had talked to Angela about the side effects of the anti-estrogen medication, but her patient had obviously not told Rob about them.

The side effects of anti-estrogen therapy are well known, and they may lead to people discontinuing the treatment.[6] *The most common side effects reported by breast cancer survivors are musculo-skeletal changes (joint stiffness and pain) and unhappiness with body image (see chapter 2). Sexual side effects include vaginal and vulvar dryness causing painful sexual touch and painful vaginal penetration (see chapter 6), as well as decreased libido*[7] *(see chapter 3).*

After Dr. Robin described the possible side effects of Angela's treatment, Rob, while not feeling better, at least felt more informed. "Thanks, Dr. Robin. I think I understand things better now. I'm still not sure why Angela hasn't shared this information with me, but we'll certainly have a talk about it, and we'll be back to see you."

"Yes, that's important," the doctor said. "Understanding is just one part of the solution. Hopefully we can talk about other suggestions that will improve things, for both of you."

Rob left Dr. Robin's office, his mind spinning with the information he'd received. He knew what he had to do, and he hoped Angela would be willing to take the next steps with him.

HENRY AND SHIRLEY

Henry, aged 70, had surgery for prostate cancer three years ago. He is married to Shirley, and, for the most part, their 40-year marriage has been a good one. They don't have children, a source of great sadness for Shirley, but she has made her peace with this. Henry's job as a police officer was one of the reasons they never had children; Shirley was always afraid Henry would be injured or worse on duty, and she didn't want to raise a child on her own. Shirley recently retired as a school librarian, and Henry retired 5 years ago at age 65.

Shirley had learned over the years of their marriage that Henry wasn't the kind of man who shared his feelings with anyone. In the early years, this frustrated her, and it was the source of many arguments. But with time, she came to accept that he wasn't going to change. She wasn't sure whether his disposition was a result of the macho culture of policing or whether it was what drew him into police work. In any event, she had come to terms with the fact that he wasn't a touchy-feely kind of man.

The road since his cancer diagnosis hadn't been easy, especially for Shirley. After the surgery to remove his prostate,

Henry found it hard to accept the loss of sexual function that he experienced. He was angry about it, and at times, he took it out on her. She'd learned over the years to not argue in response to his anger but to keep quiet and let the storm pass. Once he calmed down, he was more reasonable, and it was then that she could tell him her feelings were hurt by his words, and things would be better . . . until the next time. After the surgery, whenever he wanted to have sex but wasn't able to have an erection, his anger would shatter the calm, and nothing she did seemed to break the cycle. She thought that after months of failure to get an erection, he'd stop trying, but that didn't happen. Since going through menopause, she was quite happy for their sex life to end. In fact, she'd assumed this was expected at their age. She dared not talk to any of her friends about this; many of them were married to ex-policemen, and the thought that their troubles could get back to the other husbands was terrifying. Shirley wouldn't betray Henry by disclosing this secret, so she suffered his anger in silence.

After the cancer came back, just a year after the surgery, he had radiation therapy along with two years of androgen deprivation therapy. He'd gone alone to all his appointments, and she wasn't aware of the possible side effects of the treatment. During the eight-week course of radiation, he was tired a lot and needed to have an hour-long nap in the afternoon. He had some changes to his bowel movements, but other than that, he hadn't complained to her about any other side effects. The side effects of the androgen deprivation therapy, however, were another matter entirely.

Side effects of androgen deprivation therapy and the subsequent loss of testosterone include the following:

- *Loss of interest in sex (lowered libido)*
- *Erectile dysfunction*
- *Hot flashes*
- *Loss of bone density*
- *Bone fractures*
- *Loss of muscle mass and physical strength*
- *Changes in blood lipids*
- *Insulin resistance*
- *Weight gain*
- *Mood swings*
- *Fatigue*
- *Growth of breast tissue (gynecomastia)*[8]

Shirley had noticed differences in Henry's behavior; he was tired most of the time and had gained a lot of weight, especially around his midsection. She was nervous to say anything about it, so she tried to slowly increase the vegetables and decrease the starches in their meals. This did not go unnoticed!

"Why have you changed the food you're giving me?" he asked at supper one evening after pushing the green beans and carrots to the edge of his plate.

Shirley hesitated then replied, "I just think I need to cut down on the carbohydrates in my diet. I've put on a few pounds, and I'd like to lose them . . ." This was a lie, but she thought it could prevent an outburst from Henry.

"That's nonsense!" he responded, his voice louder than it needed to be. "You look the exact same to me, and I'm not interested in suffering because you want to lose a pound or two!"

She wondered why he hadn't noticed his clothes were tighter around his middle; she could clearly see his golf shirts were stretched, and he hadn't gone back to wearing proper pants since the radiation treatment had finished. Now he only wore sweatpants, and even they too were snug around his waist. But she knew better than to mention any of this—she'd likely get an explosion of anger from him in response.

Shirley sighed. She made a mental note to see whether she could find a cookbook at the library that might give her some ideas on how to cut calories in her cooking without Henry noticing.

He was also having night sweats, and his frequent waking meant she was getting little sleep. He soaked the sheets several times a night and woke up shivering. This of course woke her too, and she had to help him change the sheets and put on dry nightclothes. It was exhausting, and try as she might, she couldn't help being irritable the next day. And Henry was irritable too, so the result was two people on the edge of arguing all the time.

Shirley knew she had to find a way to deal with the situation, so she asked Henry whether she could go with him to his next appointment with the radiation oncologist.

"Why do you need to come with me? Don't you trust me to tell you what's going on with my health?" he grumbled.

The truth was that he didn't tell her much about what happened at these appointments, other than to say "things are going according to plan." She didn't know what the plan was or what the things were, but she didn't want to cause another argument. Now she told him she wanted to ask the oncologist about what to do about the night sweats. He wasn't keen on her talking to his doctor, but she was insistent.

Night sweats during treatment are common and range from a clammy feeling to drenching sweats that require a change of pajamas and sheets. They may come with chills, feeling warm, or a rapid heart rate.

Nonhormonal management includes these tactics:

- *Keeping the bedroom cool*
- *Wearing pajamas made of bamboo, linen, or silk*
- *Using sheets made of linen or low-thread-count percale*
- *Avoiding alcohol, caffeine, tobacco, and spicy foods*
- *Staying hydrated*
- *Maintaining a healthy weight*
- *Practicing deep breathing and meditation*
- *Trying acupuncture and doing yoga*

There are medications that might help. They aren't approved for hot flashes or night sweats, but they're prescribed off-label, and they include medications typically used to treat depression or high blood pressure. It's important to discuss these options with a health-care provider.

There is insufficient evidence to recommend the use of vitamins, minerals, and other supplements for managing night sweats or hot flashes.

While Shirley and Henry were waiting to see the oncologist at the cancer center, a nurse entered the exam room with an iPad in her hand. She asked Henry a long list of questions, which he mostly answered with a yes or no. Shirley wondered whether he was being so brief because she was with him. But once again, she didn't say anything. After about another 10 minutes, the oncologist, a man who looked too young to be a doctor never mind a specialist, came into the room, and the nurse left. Shirley followed her out; she was sure Henry didn't want her in the room while he talked to the doctor, but she hoped she would have an opportunity to join him before the appointment was over.

As she walked to the waiting room, the nurse, who'd introduced herself as Michelle, asked her how she was doing. This was the first time anyone, including her friends, had asked Shirley how she was coping.

"Oh, I guess I'm doing okay . . ." she answered tentatively. "My husband, he's tired a lot, and it's a big change from the way he used to be. He was always busy with something, and now he pretty much sits in his chair most of the day."

"Yes, most people are surprised at how tired they are," Michelle said. "At first, it's from the radiation therapy, but then the injections, the loss of testosterone, those take away that male energy that many men have." She smiled. "But that's about your husband, I was asking about the impact of your husband's cancer on *you*." The nurse emphasized the last word, and Shirley was a little shocked.

"Well, I guess I'm not used to how the cancer has changed him, you know?" she said. "He's always been pretty type A, but now, well, he's grumpy, and he flies off the handle really quickly . . ."

"Did anyone discuss with you the possible changes that men experience while on the medication?"

Shirley shook her head. "This is the only time he's allowed me to come to the cancer center . . . I wanted to talk to his doctor about the night sweats he has. They're just awful, and I'm at my wit's end."

"I can try and give you some advice about that," Michelle replied. "And I have a handout that I can give you."

"That would be great. I don't know why Henry hasn't shared anything with me."

Once she'd started talking to the nurse, Shirley found she couldn't stop. She told Michelle the thing that bothered her the most was that Henry never kissed her anymore or initiated sex. He'd always been a very sexual person, despite his increasing age, and she didn't understand why he'd stopped touching her. Once she admitted this, she realized that she'd felt lonely for the past two years and that her loneliness was only growing harder and harder to deal with.

Providing care for someone with cancer disrupts the caregiver's usual daily routines and social relationships, which can result in feeling lonely. Loneliness can negatively impact your social, emotional, and physical health.[9] *It can also lead to a feeling of hopelessness and an inability to care for yourself as well as the loved one with cancer. To address lonely feelings, try to make it a priority to reach out to your established social contacts, and to establish new friendships with others going through something similar. Attending support groups, often available through cancer centers, is a good way to do this. Reaching out to a mental health-care professional, or starting by contacting a personal physician, can help as well.*

"Do you think he's having an affair?" Shirley asked the nurse. As she said the words, she covered her mouth with her hand. She was shocked and embarrassed she'd said this to a stranger.

Michelle reached out and put her hand on Shirley's shoulder. "You have no idea how many women think that, and ask the exact same question," she said with a small smile. "In almost all cases, the lack of physical touch is related to the loss of testosterone and not because the man is having an affair. In addition, men facing erectile dysfunction after prostate surgery may not want to initiate any kind of physical touch."

Shirley gave a big sigh. She realized now just how much she'd been worried, but she'd been unable to say the words out loud. "Does this happen with all men?"

"Not all," the nurse said. "But it's common and usually causes distress for the man's partner. Have you talked to your husband about how you feel?"

"No . . . I'm not sure how he'd react."

"That's the first step. Your husband may not even be aware of this change in your relationship. I know it sounds strange, but that's how it is for many men when they have very low or no testosterone in their body."

"I had no idea. I'm really glad I talked to you," Shirley said. "Is there anything that can be done to change things?"

"Talking to your husband and describing how it feels for you is a good first step. It may help if we get one of our social workers involved. They're very helpful in facilitating difficult conversations between couples. Do you think your husband would be willing to do that?"

"Can he take some medication to fix this instead?" Shirley was pretty sure Henry wouldn't want to talk about his private life with a stranger.

"There isn't medication that would change things, but time may," Michelle said. "Once the testosterone-lowering medication is out of his system, his interest in sex may increase."

Loss of erections is common after all treatments for prostate cancer. Six months after surgery to remove the prostate, 95% of men are unable to achieve an erection[10] and just 43% of men under the age of 65 experience a return to their baseline erectile function.[11] In men who were treated with radiation, 88% experience erectile problems six months after treatment.[10] Two years after the end of testosterone-blocking treatment, about half of men see a return to sexual function, including interest in sex, as they experienced before treatment.[12] They're also two years older, however, and it's normal for testosterone levels to decrease in men as they age.

"That might help," Shirley said. "Thank you so much for the information. You've really helped a lot. Do you think I could go back to talk to the doctor about night sweats now?"

Shirley had learned enough from Michelle for the moment. There were so many thoughts swirling in her head, but she also wanted to start dealing with one practical thing—how to get a good night's sleep. Talking to Henry could come later, when they were alone at home. At least she hoped so.

CONCLUSION

Caring for someone with cancer has a significant impact on many aspects of the couple's relationship. The caregiving partner will likely take on additional responsibilities, and they'll naturally be afraid of losing someone they love. In addition, loss of sexual function as a result of the cancer itself or its treatment can interfere with the usual ways the couple expresses affection, which can lead to profound feelings of loneliness and isolation. Misunderstandings and assumptions can lead to further feelings of loneliness and even suspicion. It's important for both partners to receive accurate information about sexual side effects, and it's equally important for the couple to communicate about the changes and their impacts. The partner of the cancer survivor should address their mental, social, and emotional health alongside the survivor, so that both can receive the care they need to function well in all areas of life.

TAKEAWAYS

- Cancer is a couple's disease as the partner of the cancer patient is profoundly affected by changes in the relationship.

- Partners may ignore their own needs and put the needs of the patient before their own.

- The partner needs to ensure they're taking care of their own physical and emotional health in order to provide care for their loved one.

- Connecting with other partners in a similar situation can be a source of valuable support and coping mechanisms.

- Discussing concerns with medical and mental health-care professionals is a good first step to getting help.

WEBSITES FOR ADDITIONAL INFORMATION

For the partner of someone with breast cancer

American Cancer Society
Features information on breast cancer, treatment, and support services, including a helpline
https://www.cancer.org

Breastcancer.org
Offers comprehensive information on breast cancer, treatment options, and support resources
https://www.breastcancer.org

Living Beyond Breast Cancer

Provides programs, services, and support for everyone impacted by breast cancer

https://www.lbbc.org/family-friends

Sharsheret

Offers support for Jewish women and families facing breast cancer, including resources and community connections

https://sharsheret.org

Susan G. Komen

Provides education, support, and funding for breast cancer research, along with resources for patients and survivors

https://www.komen.org

For the partner of someone with prostate cancer

Prostate Cancer Foundation

Provides support and information for the partner of the man with prostate cancer

https://www.pcf.org/patient-resources/patient
-navigation/for-caregivers/

Zero Prostate Cancer

Provides information for partners about sex after prostate cancer

https://zerocancer.org/blog/prostate-cancer-and
-marriage-start-great-sex

Further resources for the partner

CancerCare

Provides free support services, including counseling and financial assistance for those affected by cancer

https://cancercare.org

Caregiver Action Network

Provides resources and support specifically for caregivers of individuals with chronic illnesses, including cancer

https://www.caregiveraction.org

Well Spouse Association

Offers support for spouses and partners of individuals with chronic illnesses, including cancer

https://wellspouse.org

CHAPTER 10

"I miss touching her"

Sexuality at the End of Life

The need for touch doesn't go away at the end of life; in fact, touch may be even more treasured when time left is finite. People at or near the end of life are often regarded as "untouchable," and partners may feel the need to receive permission to touch their loved one. Sexuality at the end of life is challenging; couples may be reluctant to initiate any kind of touch that may be misconstrued as sexual initiation rather than touch for connection or comfort. Health care providers may unfortunately not even consider that touch remains a need at this stage of illness.

JOE AND SARA

The past 5 years have been challenging for Joe, aged 62, and his wife, Sara, who is the same age. Like so many others, his diagnosis of cancer came as a shock, but for Joe, who owned a wine store, the diagnosis of tongue cancer seemed especially cruel. Joe not only sold wine, he loved it and had studied the science of wine for years. He'd inherited the store from his father and had turned it into a destination not just for wine lovers in their city but for many in the state. Sara wasn't as passionate about wine as Joe was, but she worked in the store and took care of the many details of inventory management and accounting.

A large part of Joe's daily life involved tasting new wines and refreshing his knowledge about well-established wineries. This work was put in jeopardy when he was told the most effective treatment for tongue cancer was surgical removal of his tongue. This would affect his ability to taste and to speak. The thought of losing these capacities was unimaginable, and Joe considered refusing treatment. But at Sara's insistence, they asked for a second opinion and were referred to a radiation oncologist who offered Joe a course of radiation therapy instead of surgery. The treatment was not going to be easy to get through, but there was a chance that he would regain his ability to taste and that his speech would be minimally affected.

Tongue cancer is a form of head and neck cancer, and it's associated with the human papilloma virus (HPV). Twice as many men are diagnosed with this cancer as women,[1] and it affects those over 45 most commonly. A history of smoking and alcohol use as well as poor oral hygiene are known risk factors.

Joe got through the weeks of radiation therapy, but it wasn't easy. He couldn't eat or drink, and the pain was awful; he wasn't able to work and had to be fed through a tube into his stomach. It took weeks for his tongue to heal and even longer for his ability to taste to return. Everything was stable for four and a half years, but then the cancer returned, and Joe made the decision to not have any more treatment. Over the following six months he and Sara closed the wine store, sold all the inventory, and took one last trip to Napa, where he spent hours staring at the vineyards. In the past, these vistas had excited him, but now they were bittersweet. He didn't want to visit any of the wineries, and even just tasting his favorite wines was painful, both physically and emotionally. They returned home after only two days—staying any longer would've been too hard for both of them.

When they returned from their trip, Joe talked to his primary care provider and requested a referral to hospice. Dr. Brice had been Joe's primary care provider for almost 20 years. She'd first noticed the white patches on his tongue and had sent him for the biopsy that had resulted in his diagnosis. She'd supported him while he'd undergone the radiation therapy and had remained in close contact with both Sara and Joe during the long weeks of his recovery. She'd also been supportive when he'd decided to forgo further treatment.

"Of course I'll make the referral for hospice," she said now. "Have you and Sara discussed whether you'd prefer home hospice or admission to a hospice facility?"

Joe and Sara hadn't discussed this, and Joe was unsure of the difference between the two kinds of care.

Dr. Brice explained that, if he opted to stay at home, he'd receive regular visits from a physician and nurse, and he'd get any other resources, such as a hospital bed, as needed. "You need to talk to Sara about this," Dr. Brice continued. "This affects her too, and her opinion should be considered."

"I don't know where to begin," Joe said. "Can you help me talk to Sara about this?"

"Of course," the doctor said. "How about the two of you come in tomorrow at the end of my clinic, and we'll talk about the options?"

"Hospice care" refers to the special services that people with terminal illness can access if their life expectancy is six months or shorter.[2] Services include pain and symptom control, and access to equipment, such as a hospital bed, oxygen, and other resources—but there's no active treatment such as chemotherapy. People who

choose hospice care experience fewer visits to emergency depart-
ments as well as increased satisfaction and better end-of-life care.[3]

Joe and Sara spent over an hour with Dr. Brice, talking about
what Joe wanted in his final days or weeks. It was a difficult conversation, but Dr. Brice coaxed them into sharing painful feelings. Sara thought Joe was giving up too soon—she still had
hope he'd live for a few more months. Joe was insistent that his
quality of life was poor, and he was afraid of a painful death and
how it would affect Sara. At the end of the discussion, Joe decided he would try home hospice, and if that didn't work out,
he would go into a hospice facility.

Dr. Brice made the referral, and within four days, they'd received a visit from the palliative care team—a physician, nurse,
and home care aide. The physician prescribed pain medication
as well as sedatives to use if Joe couldn't sleep. Over the next
few days, a variety of equipment arrived—a special stool for the
shower, a commode in case Joe had difficulty getting to the toilet, and a home oxygen machine. Sara was shocked at how
quickly their home turned into what felt like a hospital.

All the preparations, however, didn't hide the fact that Joe
was in constant pain, and Sara wasn't managing well at all. The
nights were particularly difficult; Joe moaned constantly, even
in his short periods of sleep. Sara was sleeping beside him in
their king-size bed, but the sound of him in pain meant she
got little sleep and was exhausted. She was also scared—it was
her job to give him the pain medication, and she worried she
might accidentally give him too much, causing him to stop
breathing.

At the nurse's next visit, Sara shared her fears, feeling like a
failure.

"I hear you," the nurse said softly. "How about I talk to your husband to see if he'd be willing to transfer to the hospice facility?"

Sara was grateful for the offer and relieved when Joe told her he'd decided to move to the hospice.

"Are you sure?" she asked, half-afraid he would change his mind.

"Yes, I'm sure. I don't want you to remember our bed and our home as the place where I died . . ."

Sara was surprised by his insight; that had in fact been something else she was afraid of. She loved their home and the memories of making love in their bed. The thought of Joe actually taking his last breaths there had been in the back of her mind, but she had tried to ignore it. Now it was out in the open, and she felt as if a weight had been lifted off her shoulders.

The next day Joe moved into hospice. He was given a room facing a garden with large trees. There was a queen-size bed in the room with a colorful quilt. Sara was happy to see it looked nothing like a hospital room, but Joe hardly seemed to notice. What wasn't different from a hospital, in Sara's opinion, was the constant coming and going of staff. There seemed to be an unending stream of people—staff and volunteers—checking on Joe and asking her whether she needed anything.

"What I need most is some time alone with my husband who is dying" was her thought on the situation, but she wasn't sure who to share this with. It seemed rude to say something like that, given how good Joe's care was.

An opportunity presented itself on Joe's third day at the hospice, when the nurse manager came to talk to them. She asked them if there was anything they wanted to talk about, anything they felt was missing in Joe's care.

"Um, I'm not sure how to say this . . ." Sara was hesitant to speak out. She hadn't talked to Joe about this, and she didn't want to embarrass him. "I just wish that we had more time to be alone . . ."

Joe had been resting, his eyes closed, but he now was instantly present.

"It's just that, well, I miss my husband so much . . . in that way, you know?"

Joe now looked embarrassed. He was probably wondering what she was talking about, or if he understood what she was trying to say, why she'd bring it up now. The nurse manager didn't seem at all embarrassed or confused; in fact, she seemed to know exactly what Sara meant.

The sexual needs of the person at or close to the end of life and their partner aren't always discussed with the palliative care team[4] despite these needs being seen as a fundamental part of palliative care and included in clinical practice guidelines for palliative care professionals. This omission in care is related to incorrect assumptions, both the health-care providers' and patients' or partners' discomfort with the topic, and a lack of education for health-care providers on the importance of sexual needs at or near the end of life.[5] "Sexual needs" doesn't necessarily mean sexual intercourse, which may not be possible or desirable because of physical factors,[6] but rather the term can encompass nongenital touch and verbal communication.[7]

"What I hear you saying is that you want to spend some private time with your husband," the nurse manager said, "where no one will disturb you." She nodded. "We can absolutely make sure that happens, and I'm sorry if no one has talked to you about this."

The nurse manager went on to ask whether the couple were comfortable with a sign on the outside of the door indicating they were not to be disturbed. She also suggested Joe's pain medication could be timed so he'd have maximum pain relief when they wanted to have physical contact. And finally, she asked whether Joe would be comfortable with being moved in the bed so Sara could lie next to him.

Joe wasn't sure how to respond or even whether he needed to respond. Sara had reached out to hold his hand while the nurse had been talking, and as she'd done that, he'd realized it had been ages since they'd touched, beyond when he'd needed help to get to the bathroom at home.

When someone has advanced cancer and is facing the terminal phase of the illness, the partner often becomes involved in their technical care, and their role changes from that of intimate and sexual partner to that of caregiver.[8] The partner may be afraid of causing pain with their physical touch or discomfort from the medical devices that might be supporting the person with cancer.

"I'd love that," Sara replied to the nurse's suggestion.

"Joe, can you move a little to your left or do you need some help with that?" the nurse asked.

Since moving to the hospice and receiving increasing doses of pain medication, Joe had been reluctant to move once he'd gotten into a comfortable position. But the look on Sara's face when the nurse suggested she lie next to him gave him the energy he needed to move over, even though it hurt. Sara sat gently on the edge of the bed, and with the encouragement of the nurse, she lay down carefully. She rested her arm over his chest, her head on the pillow next to his. Joe closed his eyes and sighed as he felt the weight of her arm over his body.

He didn't notice the tears that fell silently from his wife's eyes onto the pillow. The nurse covered them both with the quilt and left the room, closing the door quietly behind her.

MARG AND JANE

Marg and Jane have been a couple for 40 years, ever since they met on a blind date. They'd both been out lesbians since their early 20s and are now both 70 years old. Marg has metastatic breast cancer, and after trying an experimental treatment for her disease that failed, two months ago she accepted that there was no other treatment left. Jane has had a hard time accepting this, and for a while she tried to persuade Marg to go to Mexico for another experimental treatment, but Marg refused.

Marg had been getting weaker over the past couple of weeks and decided it was time to enroll in the palliative care program offered by the cancer clinic where she'd been treated. She didn't tell Jane immediately, but then she was forced to after she broke a rib bumping into some furniture. An X-ray showed the cancer had spread to three ribs. So Marg told Jane about her decision on the palliative care referral. Jane was alternately furious and devastated; she hated that Marg had hidden something from her, and she was floored by the reality that her beloved partner was close to the end of her life.

Now that palliative care was no longer a secret, Marg asked Jane to meet the team from the program. Jane had admitted she knew little about what palliative care meant. But she wanted to support Marg, so she was grateful for the opportunity to meet the team and learn from them.

"Palliative care" refers to pain and symptom management, and providing comfort and improving quality of life for both cancer survivors and their family caregivers. It's not dependent on the stage of illness, and it can be offered while someone continues to receive treatment for their disease.

Meeting the physician and nurse from the palliative care program was a game changer for Jane. She was relieved and grateful that they'd do their best to ensure Marg was pain-free in her last weeks and that they'd also support her. What surprised her was the speed with which Marg's health declined once Jane had met the palliative care team. Marg's condition worsened so much that within days she was unable to do even the simplest tasks for herself. She needed help going to the bathroom, and she hardly ate or drank anything.

The palliative care nurse, Mallory, visited Marg at home every day. She bathed Marg and cleaned her mouth gently with a wet swab. She changed the sheets while talking softly to her patient. Jane showered while Mallory took care of these tasks. A couple of times, Jane even managed to sit outside for 20 minutes, her face turned to the early fall sun.

Early on, Mallory suggested they arrange for a hospital bed to be set up in the living room. Their bedroom was on the second floor, and Marg couldn't manage the stairs, plus Jane was tired out from going up and down the stairs multiple times a day. Mallory also explained to Jane what a meal train was—a plan she could share with their friends who wanted to help with meals. Organizing a meal train meant food wouldn't go to waste, what with Jane's appetite gone and the fridge already full of casseroles and sandwiches.

Another problem was that Jane was becoming overwhelmed with the number of well-meaning friends who popped in at all hours to help. They mostly sat around the dining room table, and Jane found herself constantly making tea and coffee, and then having to clean up after they'd left. After just two days of this, Jane was exhausted. She wasn't sleeping well alone in their bed upstairs, and she couldn't get to sleep on the couch in the living room, next to the hospital bed where Marg lay.

While many people would rather die at home than in hospital, it's not always easy for family members to facilitate this. The family or other caregivers need to be supported practically (help with meals, laundry, etc.), mentally (managing medication schedules safely), and emotionally (knowing what to expect in the final days and hours). For family members, the benefits of having the dying loved one at home include a sense of purpose, fulfilling the wishes of the dying person, and being with them so they're not alone. But witnessing the death of a loved one can be emotionally upsetting, and, in the short or long term, there is the risk that the caregiver's home becomes a trigger for grief and loss rather than a sanctuary.[9]

Once again, Mallory's advice was invaluable. With Jane's permission, Barb, Marg's best friend since their teen years, was tasked with creating a visitors' log so that people arrived at designated times and had assigned jobs. This gave Jane some quiet time to rest, and it helped with getting the laundry and cleaning done so Jane could focus on Marg rather than household chores.

Marg slept most of the time now, whether because of the effects of the pain medication or as part of the dying process.

Jane admitted to Mallory that she was terrified Marg would die when the nurse wasn't there.

"How will I know that she's gone?" Jane asked, tears filling her eyes. "How will I know that she . . . you know . . . is close to . . . the end?"

Jane was sobbing now, her hands covering her eyes. They were in the kitchen, and it was one of Jane's "rest times" when no one else was there.

Mallory sat quietly while Jane cried. She knew Jane would stop eventually, and Mallory would then be able to explain what was likely to happen in Marg's final hours and minutes. Jane did stop crying, and her eyes widened as she focused on what Mallory started to explain.

"If you don't think you can manage," Mallory said, "there is always the option of moving Marg to the palliative care unit at the hospital."

"Oh no! I couldn't do that! What if they won't let me be with her? I've heard stories about how gay couples have been treated in hospitals!" Jane was crying again.

Despite improvements in palliative care for cancer survivors, barriers exist for sexual minority (gay, lesbian, bisexual, or trans) survivors and their partners or spouses. Health-care providers report they've observed instances where care for these individuals or couples was disrespectful (15.6%), and where care was inadequate (7.3%) or even abusive (1.6%); in addition, 43% reported instances of discrimination toward the patient's partner or spouse.[10] Older lesbians may be at increased risk due to vulnerability to isolation and poverty.[9] Barriers to palliative care include homophobia and discrimination as well as mistrust of health-care providers.[11]

Mallory tried to calm Jane, but she wasn't entirely successful. She'd also heard the stories of gay and lesbian couples being treated horribly, but in her experience, times had changed, and she hoped those prejudices and outdated policies were in the past.

Mallory had also noticed something else. Jane appeared to be hesitant to touch Marg, perhaps out of fear of causing her pain, or perhaps she just didn't know what to do. Mallory was aware that Jane was almost always absent when she bathed Marg, and she wondered whether this was intentional or because Jane didn't feel she had permission to be engaged in Marg's personal care.

"Jane, I'm going to bathe Marg in a few minutes," Mallory said. "I could do with some help . . ."

Jane was surprised by Mallory's request. She'd always been hesitant to ask the nurse, who was so competent and efficient, whether she needed help. But the invitation right now seemed perfect. "I'd love to," she said, "if you could show me what to do."

"Why don't you sit with Marg while I gather the supplies," Mallory said. "I bet she'd love to hear your voice."

Although the need or ability to participate in sexual activity may wane in the terminal stages of illness, the need for touch and connectedness does not necessarily fade. For those in hospital or another institution, the only touch experienced may be from gloved hands. People may suffer from the absence of loving and intimate touch in the final months, weeks, or days of life, and if health-care providers don't recognize and deal with this, they're doing their patients a disservice.

The two women then bathed Marg as she lay in bed, seemingly asleep but with a small smile on her lips. Mallory showed

Jane how to gently wipe a warm washcloth over her partner's limbs. Mallory tuned Marg from side to side as Jane quietly cleaned Marg's back and then chest, her hand shaking as she passed over the left side where Marg's breast used to be. Jane hadn't realized how thin Marg was; it had been weeks since she'd seen Marg's naked body, and she was shocked at the change. Marg's skin was almost translucent, and when Mallory offered a bottle of lotion to Jane, she hesitated before taking some, but then she gently massaged the sweet-smelling lotion into Marg's hands and arms.

Jane was humming quietly now but seemed unaware she was doing so. Mallory recognized a Joni Mitchell song and then one that might've been from Simon and Garfunkel, but she wasn't sure. What she was sure of was that Jane was physically present but mentally somewhere else, and Mallory didn't want to disturb her or Marg.

The nurse noticed Marg's breathing had slowed, and then it stopped. But she didn't say anything. There was time enough to let Jane know that Marg was no longer with them, but this wasn't yet the moment.

CONCLUSION

While talking about the end of life is difficult for many, it's important to acknowledge this final stage of living with cancer; it shouldn't be shrouded in secrecy, nor does it need to be the end of physical contact. Certainly, the end of life brings with it many unknowns for spouses or partners and other family members. But an important aspect of this stage is that the need for loving touch doesn't go away, even in the final hours and minutes of life. Loving touch doesn't mean sexual touch, but spouses or partners may still need permission to be close to their loved one at this time. Although some may hesitate, many people find having physical contact with their dying loved one is a rewarding and special experience.

TAKEAWAYS

- Sexuality at or near the end of life usually doesn't include sexual intercourse.
- If intercourse is something both partners are interested in, even at the end of life, accommodations can sometimes be made in concert with health-care personnel.
- Human touch without gloves is essential at this time.
- Facilitating the death of a loved one at home isn't always possible despite one's best efforts.
- Hospice care can be provided at home or in special units or institutions.
- Palliative care is the process of providing pain and symptom management and isn't about "giving up" on life.
- Having personal time alone for physical contact can be a rewarding part of the dying process for both partners.
- Helping a health-care provider such as a nurse or aide to bathe a loved one at or near the end of life can be a source of comfort to both the dying person and their spouse or partner.

WEBSITES FOR ADDITIONAL INFORMATION

Cancer.Net (video on palliative care)
https://www.youtube.com/watch?v=eUaU6S-Dtlw

CaringInfo
https://www.caringinfo.org

Meal Train (how to organize meals for a friend or family member)
https://www.mealtrain.com

National Institute on Aging (NIH) (video on palliative care and hospice care)
https://www.youtube.com/watch?v=BteIA1kUizE

CHAPTER 11

Communication

Good communication lies at the heart of a healthy sex life, but it's often difficult to achieve between partners, especially at the beginning of a new relationship, when illness brings unexpected changes, and when partners need to speak with health-care providers about changes in sexual function.

This chapter offers guidance on how to start the conversation with your partner about how things have changed for you. It also describes strategies for talking with health-care providers who may seem reluctant to address these issues.

WHY IS IT SO HARD (FOR MANY PEOPLE) TO TALK ABOUT SEX?

Many people find it hard to talk about sex with their partner, their children, or health-care providers. Sex is used to sell products and as a source of jokes and teasing, but having a serious conversation about it is a source of embarrassment. There are many reasons for this, starting with our family of origin where talking about sex and even body parts may have been a taboo. Some of us learned about sex from books, TV, and movies where the depictions of people talking about sex included lots innuendo and not much honest discussion using correct names for body parts. Sexual activity is most often portrayed as a well-orchestrated dance between two (or more) people where nothing goes "wrong"; no weird noises are heard, and the people involved have "perfect" bodies and are almost always young and beautiful. There are no wrinkles, saggy breasts or abdomens, scars or missing body parts, and mutual mind-blowing orgasms are the norm. Things happen spontaneously, there are no awkward moments, and no one talks or tells their partner what to do or where to touch them. This is far from real life!

Society also has inaccurate views on sexuality more generally and who is sexual. Many people assume that women have lower sex drives than men and that people of all genders who are older than 50 no longer desire sex. These notions and assumptions are not true. Research on a community sample of older adults shows that, while sexual activity declines with age, both men and to a lesser extent women continue to be sexually active, alone or with a partner, into their 70s and 80s.[1] The most common reasons for sexual activity to end are the absence of a partner or illness in either partner.

Add to these misconceptions the societal messages that promote the myths that "nice" girls shouldn't want to have sex and that men want it all the time. Most sex education, if it exists at all, focuses on the menstrual cycle for girls and wet dreams for boys. Some programs might focus on abstinence, and others might or might not include discussions of birth control or the prevention of sexually transmitted infections. In more recent times, the focus of school-based sex education has been on consent, which is a good thing, but nothing is mentioned about pleasure and communication beyond saying no. Masturbation is still regarded by many as a sin or "less than" sex and not as something that helps us learn what feels good so that we can tell a partner what brings us pleasure. Surely, few or none of the programs focus on what a healthy sex life might look like.

And then there is the fear many people have that if they tell their partner what they want and need, they'll hurt their partner's feelings or offend them. But how is a new partner to know what brings us pleasure if we don't use our words to describe how or where we want to be touched, or whether we want to be touched at all? Despite having the gift of words and the ability to communicate, we humans often communicate like dolphins and whales, with grunts and squeaks, assuming our partner understands those sounds.

All of this gets more complicated when our sexuality—which includes desire, arousal, response, and body image—is disrupted by cancer or its treatments. It can be difficult to explain to your partner that what used to be pleasurable is now painful, numb, or unwanted. They may continue to use the same touch that's worked for months or years without realizing our response is now different or absent. But if we don't explain this, they'll continue, and as time goes on, we'll find it more and more difficult to tell them what doesn't work anymore.

HOW TO TALK TO YOUR PARTNER ABOUT SEX

Like any sensitive topic, it's important to first think about what you want to say to your partner. This isn't a subject to talk about when you're tired or cranky, after an unsuccessful attempt at sexual activity, or when you're rushing to work or an appointment. Here are some more tips to get ready:

- Plan *where* you're going to talk about sex. This isn't a discussion for the bedroom!

- Find a neutral place to talk where you won't be disturbed.

- The TV and phones should be turned off and other distractions minimized.
- Speak plainly and avoid euphemisms that can be misunderstood.
- Talk in "I" statements ("I like it when you touch my X" instead of "You don't touch me the way I like").
- Avoid statements that are blaming ("You want to have sex all the time" can be better phrased as "I want to have sex less than you do since my treatment").
- Clarify what you've heard and ask your partner what they've understood from what you've said.
- Allow time and space for your partner to ask questions or comment—they're part of the solution—and *listen* to what they have to say.
- When your partner is talking, try to avoid thinking about what you'll say in response; getting ready to respond prevents you from actively listening.
- Be flexible if your partner has a different perspective; seeing things differently doesn't mean they're wrong.
- Accept that the conversation may be awkward at first, but it will get easier.
- Remember to breathe!
- It's possible you'll address all your concerns, thoughts, and feelings in one conversation, but it's more likely that parts of the discussion will take place over time. As your sex life resumes or evolves, if it does, your concerns may decrease.
- Talking to a health-care provider can be helpful, and you can address any issues that come up as you resume sexual activity.

TALKING TO HEALTH-CARE PROVIDERS

Cancer survivors may be reluctant to talk about changes to their sexuality or sexual functioning with their health-care providers. Patients may think their provider is embarrassed or reluctant to talk about sexual concerns,[2] or they wait for the health-care provider to initiate the conversation, but when this doesn't happen, patients don't ask questions or raise their concerns. This is especially true of older patients,[3] who've been shown to be reluctant to ask questions or seek help; and if the health-care provider doesn't initiate a conversation about changes to sexuality, patients assume it's not important. Research shows that information about sexual changes after cancer is an unmet need for more than 25% of cancer survivors.[4] The information needs of sexual and gender minorities (gay, lesbian, bisexual, and transgender people) is a specific unmet necessity.[5]

Talking about sex is especially difficult for health-care providers treating adolescent and younger adults.[6] The parent of the young person may be uncomfortable talking about sex, and the young patient may be reluctant to ask any questions when the parent is present at appointments. Health-care providers often want to avoid embarrassing patients, and a young person may seem embarrassed by discussions about sexuality and sexual activity.

We live in an ageist society, and health-care providers, like the general public, may assume a patient is too old to be sexually active. This assumption isn't supported by the evidence,[1] which suggests people remain sexually active, in one form or another, into the 70s and beyond. It's also commonly thought that single people aren't sexually active, and even that women beyond childbearing years are no longer sexual!

Health-care providers may also find it difficult to talk to their patients[7] because of a lack of knowledge in their own professional education,[8] or because of a fear of offending the patient[9] or of seeming to pry or otherwise intrude on the personal lives of their patients if they ask about something so private. And health-care providers sometimes have the same hang-ups as their patients when it comes to embarrassing themselves or blushing! Oncology care providers and associated staff have a responsibility to advise patients about *all* the side effects of the treatments they recommend—and that includes the sexual side effects.

Another barrier for oncology care providers is the assumption that talking about the sexual side effects of treatment takes too much time and will disrupt the flow of patient care in busy clinics.[10] It's sometimes assumed that asking about sexuality or sexual functioning is going to lead to a long and involved therapy session. In reality, what patients want is validation that any changes they're experiencing are common, expected, and normal given their diagnosis and treatment. They'll often find the offer of support to be a relief. In addition, healthy sexual function and activity, however each patient may define that personally, contributes to overall wellbeing and should be part of every treatment plan.

To ensure your questions or concerns are addressed by your health-care provider, you can do the following:[11]

- Tell your health-care provider you have questions about sexuality or sexual functioning and would like a separate appointment if necessary to discuss them.
- Don't worry that you don't know the "correct" or medical term for what you're experiencing; use words you're comfortable with.

- Ask about the sexual side effects you should anticipate from any treatment. You can phrase your question like this: "How will X affect my sex life?"

- If your health-care provider doesn't have helpful answers for any questions you have, ask whether there's someone else you can talk to about your problems. There may be a nurse, social worker, sex therapist, or counselor in the hospital or cancer center.

- You can also ask for a referral to a sex therapist or counselor. If you're already working with a mental health provider, bring your concerns up in those sessions as well.

GETTING PROFESSIONAL HELP

There is much confusion about what actually happens during sex therapy or counseling. Some people think they have to have intercourse or masturbate in front of the therapist, or they assume a physical exam is part of the process. This isn't true!

Sex therapy or counseling is a form of talk therapy that helps the client with the emotional and mental aspects of sex-related issues. The therapist/counselor provides a safe and nonjudgmental environment for the client to explore what's causing them anxiety or distress. The therapist/counselor suggests strategies to address their problems and to enhance communication with their intimate partner(s). The client can then practice these strategies by doing homework and reflective exercises.

The therapist/counselor may see the individual alone for a first appointment or the couple together, with separate appointments at a later date. Every therapist/counselor has their own way of practicing, and while there is variation in their approaches, there is never nudity involved!

Therapists/counselors have been trained to be empathetic and to make the conversation as comfortable as possible for the client. Like in any relationship, however, you may not mesh well with one particular therapist, and you shouldn't be afraid to say you want to find someone else to provide this service or support. Some people find they prefer a therapist/counselor who's the same sex as they are, and it's your choice to see whoever you're most comfortable with. There are some therapists who work in tandem with another therapist of the opposite sex. There are also gay, lesbian, bisexual, or transgender therapists who specialize in these specific populations.

Most therapists encourage couples to talk to each other during an appointment by asking probing questions and then listening to the conversation, interrupting gently if things start to get heated. They'll often ask clients to incorporate sensual touch exercises (see appendix 2) as homework between sessions or suggest books to read. You can find a list of suggested books in chapter 13.

Other professionals who may provide support include urologists, gynecologists, and sexual medicine specialists. These are all medical practitioners, and while they can prescribe medications, such as pills for erectile problems or hormone therapies for vaginal dryness, they usually don't provide in-depth therapy or counseling. The therapist/counselor, unless they're a licensed medical practitioner with authority to prescribe, will not prescribe medication or tell the client to stop taking a medication that has been prescribed. The therapist/counselor may, with the client's permission, communicate with a health-care provider to suggest interventions that are beyond the scope of the therapist's practice. Chapter 13 also lists associations that offer online information about therapists/counselors by city and state.

CONCLUSION

Cancer treatments cause sexual difficulties for many survivors; there's no one to blame for this, and often you'll have to adapt to the new you as an individual and part of a couple. If your oncologist hasn't gone over the sexual side effects of your diagnosis and treatment, try not to be afraid to ask. Many sexual problems can be partly solved by talking to your partner, sometimes with the help of a professional. Talking openly and honestly about your feelings, and listening to your partner with curiosity and compassion, is often the first step in overcoming the challenges you're facing. Sometimes it's the only step! But when more is needed, consult with your health-care team, and engage the help of mental and sexual health professionals when necessary. It may not be easy to talk about sex, but when problems occur, keeping silent will only make communication more difficult and won't help to resolve any issues. Remember, if you're thinking about it, chances are your partner is too, and with good communication, solid and helpful information from professionals, and assistance when necessary, you can reestablish your sex life in a healthy and satisfying way.

ARTICLES FOR ADDITIONAL INFORMATION

"Our Favorite Relationship Advice of 2024, So Far," by Jancee Dunn and Catherine Pearson, *The New York Times* https://www.nytimes.com/2024/07/03/well/family /best-relationship-advice.html?region=BELOW_MAIN _CONTENT&block=storyline_flex_guide_recirc& name=styln-relationships&variant=show&pgtype =Article

"Which Couples Are Better at Sexual Communication?," by Elyakim Kislev, *Psychology Today* https://www.psychologytoday.com/us/blog/happy -singlehood/202002/which-couples-are-better-sexual -communication

"Sexual Communication: The Bedrock to Make Your Bed Rock," by Laurie Mintz, *Psychology Today* https://www.psychologytoday.com/us/blog/stress-and -sex/201712/sexual-communication-the-bedrock-make -your-bed-rock

"The Best Sex Advice Might Also Be the Hardest to Follow," by Catherine Pearson, *The New York Times* https://www.nytimes.com/2024/05/17/well/family/sex -intimacy-couples.html?u2g=i&unlocked_article_code =1.vk0.0Xow.cB3VzHooTH1k&smid=url-share

"Why Do Loving Couples Struggle with Sexual Communication?," by Uzma Rehman, *Psychology Today* https://www.psychologytoday.com/us/blog/lets-talk -intimacy/202002/why-do-loving-couples-struggle -sexual-communication

"Authenticity in Sexual Expression and Communication," by Judy Scheel, *Psychology Today*
https://www.psychologytoday.com/us/blog/sex-is-a
-language/202309/authenticity-in-sexual-expression
-and-communication

CHAPTER 12

Lotions, Pills, and Potions

What products can help individuals and couples experiencing sexual difficulties? Are there effective medications or remedies that can help cancer survivors with the sexual problems they experience?

This chapter describes evidence-based interventions that may help to alleviate the many sexual side effects caused by cancer treatment. It's important to discuss any intervention with a trusted member of your oncology or health-care team before trying something recommended by a friend, website, or influencer! Not all interventions are risk-free, and some may be harmful if used incorrectly.

INTERVENTIONS FOR WOMEN

There is a general lack of research about interventions for women with cancer who have sexual problems related to either the cancer or its treatments. The best evidence we have is in regard to alleviating pain with penetration (in medical terms, "dyspareunia"). There are few interventions for loss of sexual interest, or altered or absent orgasms.

Painful Penetration

Painful vaginal penetration (dyspareunia) in women treated for cancer is usually associated with loss of estrogen (because of removal of the ovaries, radiation to the pelvis, chemotherapy, or anti-estrogen medication) and the resultant thinning of the tissues of the vulva and vagina. This is now called the "genito-urinary syndrome of menopause" (GSM) rather than "vulvovaginal atrophy," as it was previously known. Management in a stepped manner is recommended.

1. MOISTURIZERS AND LUBRICANTS

Moisturizers are used for daily comfort and can be applied to the external genitalia (vulva) and/or vagina. Moisturizers are designed to adhere to and rehydrate the tissues. They do not contain hormones and are available over the counter without a prescription. The most effective products contain *hyaluronic acid* and have been shown to be as effective as local estrogen for some women.[1] Moisturizers need to be used two or three times a week and applied at night to promote absorption. You should take care to avoid moisturizers that contain parabens, glycerin, glycols, nonoxynol-9, or chlorhexidine. These irritants are included in the ingredient list on the product packaging or label. Moisturizers are not designed to be used for penetration.

Examples of moisturizers include Gynatrof, Hyalo Gyn, Revaree, and RepaGyn.

Lubricants are designed to increase comfort with vaginal penetration or sexual touch. There are different kinds of lubricants:

a) Water-based: These are entry-level products, and a wide selection is available at drugstores and online. They're cheaper than silicone-based lubricants and need to be reapplied frequently during use as they tend to dry out quickly.

Examples of water-based lubricants include Liquid Silk, Sliquid, Slippery Stuff, Yes, and Good Clean Love.

b) Silicone-based: These are more effective for women treated for cancer and will have words with the suffix "-cone" in the list of ingredients, which should be short and contain only one or two items. Silicone-based lubricants remain slick longer than water-based ones, and they're usually more expensive. They may be more difficult to find in drugstores but are available online. Silicone-based lubricants shouldn't be used with silicone dilators or sex toys as they degrade the silicone coating on these devices.

Astroglide Silicone, Überlube, and Pjur Eros are examples of silicone-based lubricants.

c) Hybrid: These lubricants contain both silicone and ingredients found in water-based lubricants, such as hyaluronic acid.

Sliquid Silk and Sutil are examples in this category of lubricants.

Note: Oil-based lubricants should not be used for vaginal penetration. In addition, food-grade oils (e.g., coconut or olive oil) should not be used in the vagina—they disrupt the pH of the vagina and lead to overgrowth of "bad" bacteria, causing irritation and infections. It's also important to avoid any products that claim to be warming, cooling, or intensifying, or products that are flavored, as these also contain irritants.

2. DILATORS AND PELVIC FLOOR PHYSIOTHERAPY

After trying moisturizers and lubricants, you can consider physical interventions.

Dilators can be used to prevent shortening and narrowing of the vagina in women treated with pelvic radiation. Adhering to ongoing use of these devices is low, and some women are reluctant to use them as they regard them as sex toys.[2] Dilators should be used two to three times a week for 5 to 10 minutes, for an indefinite period of time.[3] Clear instructions from a professional like a radiation oncologist, radiation therapist, or nurse is essential to prevent damage to the tissues.

Pelvic floor physiotherapy may be useful for women who experience pain with penetration. The muscles of the pelvic floor contract and tighten in response to pain with penetration as a protective mechanism; a combination of manual therapy, exercises, as well as education and home practice, have been shown to be effective in managing this.[4] Merely tightening these muscles (traditionally called "Kegel exercises") without education about how to do this correctly may cause harm or, at the very least, be ineffective.

It's important to seek the assistance of specialty-trained physiotherapists; the American Board of Physical Therapy Specialties (https://www.aptapelvichealth.org/ptlocator) has a directory of trained practitioners you can search by location.

Energy-based devices such as lasers (e.g., the MonaLisa Touch, Revive) have not been established as useful for women with cancer, and you should take caution in using these devices. The FDA issued a warning about them in 2018. There are no long-term studies on safety and effectiveness in the cancer population, and they're expensive.[5]

3. MIND-BODY INTERVENTIONS

Mindfulness-based meditation has been shown to help reduce pain with penetration. It's a practice that focuses on attention to the present moment in a nonjudgmental and compassionate way.[6,7] Mindfulness meditation can help alleviate stress, which may help women with pain from penetrative sex. It requires consistent practice, but it can be done at just about any time, including during sexual activity to stay present in the moment and to focus on pleasurable sensations rather than being anxious about possible pain.

Multiple easy-to-find websites and apps provide guided mindfulness meditations of various lengths. These include Headspace, Calm, Insight Timer, Balance, MindSpa, and many more. See chapter 13 for more suggestions.

4. PHARMACEUTICAL INTERVENTIONS

a) Low-dose estrogen: Low-dose local estrogen can help to thicken the tissues of the vulva and vagina, making sexual touch and vaginal penetration less painful. There is concern among many oncologists, however, that hormonal management of painful penetration in women with breast cancer may increase the risk of recurrence;[8] as a result, many physicians refuse to prescribe local estrogen for women with a history of breast cancer.[9] But there is increasing evidence that low-dose local estradiol (e.g., Vagifem, Imvexxy) is safe for women with breast cancer who are postmenopausal.[10] To make an informed decision, it's essential to have a comprehensive discussion about the benefits and risks for you in using this intervention.

b) Ospemifene: This is a selective estrogen receptor modulator (SERM), similar to tamoxifen, in oral form that's taken daily. It acts like natural estrogen on the vulvar and vaginal tissues, but it doesn't increase the risk of breast cancer recurrence. It's been shown to help manage pain with penetration, and it comes with some side effects (hot flashes, muscle spasms, and vaginal discharge)[11] but no increase in breast cancer recurrence.[12]

c) Dehydroepiandrosterone (DHEA): The use of this medication (prasterone) has been shown to be more effective than local estrogen in managing pain with penetration,[13] and it may be safer for women on aromatase inhibitors as it doesn't raise blood levels of estrogen.[14]

Loss of Sexual Interest

Loss of libido may occur after a cancer diagnosis itself or because of side effects from treatment (for example, painful sexual touch or penetration), changes in body image, anxiety and depression, or as a side effect of medication to treat mental health concerns.

Nonpharmaceutical interventions such as mindfulness-based meditation[15] and mindfulness-based sex therapy[16] have been shown to help low or absent libido. Cognitive behavioral therapy (CBT)[17] and sex therapy[18] have also been shown to be effective in restoring sexual interest.

There are no FDA-approved medications for low desire in women with cancer, although off-label use is common.[19] Testosterone, flibanserin (Addyi), and bremelanotide (Vyleesi) have been studied in premenopausal women who don't have a history of cancer,[20] but there is no evidence of safety or effectiveness in women with a history of any kind of cancer.

Altered or Absent Orgasms

There is very limited research addressing changes in or the absence of orgasms in women with cancer.

Vibrators may help. They can be purchased online or at adult stores, but increasingly, retail outlets such as Target, Walmart, and Sephora are carrying these devices. Some vibrators are intended for internal use and others for external use. They're usually made of plastic and may be covered in silicone. Vibrators may be charged with a battery, a USB, or electrical wire. They should be cleaned with soap and water after each use and stored in a cool, dry place. Clitoral vibrators, such as the Eros device (https://www.eros-therapy.com), which is FDA approved, may be especially effective.

Stopping medications that have a negative impact on orgasms, such as selective serotonin reuptake inhibitors (SSRIs) used to treat depression or anxiety, may help to restore women's orgasms,[21] but this must only be done after a discussion about the potential impact on mental health.

INTERVENTIONS FOR MEN

Most of the interventions for sexual problems in men with cancer address erectile dysfunction (ED) as a side effect of treatment for prostate cancer. Erectile dysfunction occurs in men with colorectal and bladder cancer too, and both surgery and radiation therapy to the pelvis have negative effects. Loss of libido, however, is another problem for men; this may occur as a reaction to difficulties with erections or to body-image changes (e.g., due to testicular or breast cancer), or it may occur as a result of hormonal changes from treatment for a variety of cancers (e.g., brain cancer, prostate cancer). Changes in the sensation of orgasm or pain with orgasm is another problem that needs intervention. Urine leakage with arousal or orgasm is another sexual problem that's rarely discussed. This is called "climacturia" and is distressing to men and their partners.

Erectile Dysfunction

1. PHARMACEUTICAL AGENTS

Pills are the first step in managing loss of or difficulty maintaining erections, and these include sildenafil (Viagra), tadalafil (Cialis), vardenafil (Levitra), and avanafil (Stendra).[22] These medications require a prescription from a physician or nurse practitioner, who will take a complete medication history to ensure they're safe for you to use with other medications.

A suppository inserted into the penis with an applicator (MUSE™) is marginally effective,[23] but may not be available in all locations. The suppository contains a medication that causes blood to be drawn into the penis and is known to cause stinging in the penis. It also requires a prescription, but it's an option for men who can't take any of the oral medications mentioned above.

Injecting medication (called Trimix or Bimix) into the side of the penis is highly effective in causing an erection,[24] especially for those who can't take the oral medications or for whom the pills don't work. Some men are resistant to the idea of injecting themselves, especially in the penis, but it is a very effective treatment used only when the man wants to have an erection, and it has a purely local effect (that is, no systemic effects on the rest of the body). The erection that's achieved lasts for about 45 minutes, depending on the dose. The medication can be purchased online or through a compounding pharmacy with a prescription from a licensed medical provider. Instructions on how to inject it can be found on YouTube (https://www.youtube.com/watch?v=-KGLryQMdsk).

2. PHYSICAL INTERVENTIONS

The penile pump (also called a "vacuum device") is a mechanical device that pulls blood into the penis.[25] These devices can be purchased online or at adult sex stores. Men who aren't able to take the oral medications or don't want to use penile injections may be interested in using this device.

The lubricated penis is inserted into the plastic tube of the pump, and the pump is engaged, either by hand or automatically if the pump is battery operated. A tight constriction band needs to be placed at the base of the penis to trap the blood in the penis. The constriction band can only be in place for 30 minutes as it prevents blood from reaching the skin of the penis, which will feel cold when the band is in place. Once the constriction band is removed, the blood will leave the inner tissues of the penis, and the penis will deflate.

3. SURGICAL INTERVENTION

Despite high satisfaction rates, surgery to insert a penile implant is usually the intervention of last resort[26] when none of the other interventions (pills, pump, or injections) work or are acceptable to the man. Modern penile implants are made up of three parts: A reservoir filled with saline fluid is implanted in the abdomen, and this is connected to a small pump and release valve placed in the scrotum. The reservoir is connected to two silicone cylinders placed down the length of the penis. When the man wants to have an erection, he engages the pump, which allows the saline to flow from the reservoir into the two cylinders in the penis. The erection obtained lasts until the man presses the release valve in his scrotum and the saline flows back into the reservoir.

4. PENILE REHABILITATION

Using oral medications, penile pumps, or penile injections two to three times weekly starting soon after cancer treatment may improve the quality or return of erections,[27,28] but adherence to the protocols for penile rehabilitation is low, with 55% of men experiencing a lack of progress, and so they stop.[29]

5. NEW OR EXPERIMENTAL TREATMENTS

Newer treatments such as low-intensity extracorporeal shock-wave therapy (Li-ESWT), stem cell therapy, and platelet-rich plasma [30] are available, but there is limited evidence they work for men who have been treated for cancer.[31] These treatments may be available from urologists or as part of a clinical trial, but you should be cautious if these experimental treatments are advertised as a "sure thing" as there isn't yet strong evidence for their use.

Loss of Libido

Other than supplemental testosterone therapy, which is contraindicated in men on androgen deprivation therapy, there is no other pharmaceutical treatment for loss of sexual interest. Testosterone has been used for many years to improve sexual desire in healthy men, and it can be prescribed for men other than those being treated with testosterone-blocking medications.

Mind-body interventions such as cognitive behavioral therapy or mindfulness meditation have not been shown to be effective for men with physical or hormonal causes of loss of sexual interest. But stress can impact libido, so reducing stress may help in recovering libido. Mindfulness meditation may help reduce some of the stress surrounding diagnosis and treatment and thus have a protective impact on sexual desire.

Educating the man and his sexual partner about the impact of testosterone loss on the relationship and maintaining physical contact of a nonsexual nature may be helpful.[31] It's also important for the couple to actively mourn the loss of interest and acknowledge the consequences of it on their sexual relationship. Doing so can help them move forward into a new way of connecting both physically and emotionally.[32]

Altered or Absent Sensations or Pain with Orgasm

The use of a vibrator on the penile shaft may increase the sensation of orgasms for men who experience muted or absent orgasms. Painful orgasms may be a result of pelvic-floor-muscle dysfunction, and a referral to a pelvic floor physiotherapist may be helpful. The physiotherapist can teach the man to do pelvic floor exercises that help to relax the pelvic floor muscles, reducing the pain experienced with orgasm.

Climacturia

Men may experience urine leakage, especially after removal of the prostate. This leakage can happen at any time, but it can be particularly frustrating during arousal or orgasm (called "climacturia").

Pelvic floor physiotherapy[33] and using a condom for intercourse have been suggested as a way to manage urine leakage. A constriction band at the base of the erect penis may also help.[34] Constriction bands (commonly called "cock rings") can be purchased online or from adult sex stores. Once the penis is erect, the man tightens the constriction band at the base of the penis, which traps blood in the penis, similar to the effect of the penile pump.

CONCLUSION

Sexual problems are distressing for many couples, and help is available, but the person with cancer or their partner has to ask for help. Some couples, or one of the individuals in the couple relationship, may not want help—they may be content to live without an active sex life. But there are treatments that can help. Being open to these interventions and learning how they work may be the first steps in moving toward a rewarding, if different, sex life.

CHAPTER 13

Finding Help

As with any disorder or health issue, you can find copious resources about cancer both online and in libraries and bookstores. Here is a list of resources to get you started.

BOOKS ABOUT COUPLE RELATIONSHIPS AND SEXUALITY

The Rough Patch: Marriage and the Art of Living Together, by Daphne de Marneffe

Prostate Cancer and the Man You Love, (2nd edition) by Anne Katz

Woman Cancer Sex, (2nd edition) by Anne Katz

So Tell Me About the Last Time You Had Sex: Laying Bare and Learning to Repair Our Love Lives, by Ian Kerner

Magnificent Sex: Lessons from Extraordinary Lovers, by Peggy J. Kleinplatz and A. Dana Ménard

Tell Me What You Want: The Science of Sexual Desire and How It Can Help You Improve Your Sex Life, by Justin J. Lehmiller

Enhancing Couple Sexuality, by Barry McCarthy and Emily McCarthy

Finding Your Sexual Voice: Celebrating Female Sexuality, by Barry McCarthy and Emily J. McCarthy

Enduring Desire: Your Guide to Lifelong Intimacy, by Michael E. Metz and Barry W. McCarthy

Saving Your Sex Life: A Guide for Men with Prostate Cancer, by John P. Mulhall

Come as You Are, by Emily Nagoski

Come Together, by Emily Nagoski

Mating in Captivity: Unlocking Erotic Intelligence, by Esther Perel

Happy Together: Using the Science of Positive Psychology to Build Love That Lasts, by Suzann Pileggi Pawelski and James O. Pawelski

Better Than I Ever Expected: Straight Talk About Sex After Sixty, by Joan Price

Naked at Our Age, by Joan Price

Love Worth Making: How to Have Ridiculously Great Sex in a Long-Lasting Relationship, by Stephen Snyder

Androgen Deprivation Therapy: An Essential Guide for Prostate Cancer Patients and Their Loved Ones, (3rd edition) by Richard J. Wassersug, Lauren M. Walker, and John W. Robinson

The Sex-Starved Marriage: Boosting Your Marriage Libido: A Couple's Guide, by Michele Weiner Davis

Feeling Good About the Way You Look: A Program for Overcoming Body Image Problems, by Sabine Wilhelm

Gay and Bisexual Men Living with Prostate Cancer, by Jane M. Ussher, Janette Perz, and B. R. Simon Rosser

BOOKS ABOUT MINDFULNESS

Radical Acceptance: Embracing Your Life with the Heart of a Buddha, by Tara Brach

Better Sex Through Mindfulness: How Women Can Cultivate Desire, by Lori A. Brotto

Mindfulness-Based Cancer Recovery, by Linda E. Carlson and Michael Speca

Falling Awake: How to Practice Mindfulness in Everyday Life, by Jon Kabat-Zinn

Full Catastrophe Living: Using the Wisdom of Your Body and Mind to Face Stress, Pain, and Illness, (revised edition) by Jon Kabat-Zinn

The Healing Power of Mindfulness: A New Way of Being, by Jon Kabat-Zinn

Meditation Is Not What You Think: Mindfulness and Why It Is So Important, by Jon Kabat-Zinn

Mindfulness for Beginners: Reclaiming the Present Moment—and Your Life, by Jon Kabat-Zinn

Wherever You Go, There You Are: Mindfulness Meditation in Everyday Life, by Jon Kabat-Zinn

Self-Compassion: The Proven Power of Being Kind to Yourself, by Kristin Neff

The Art of Mindfulness: A Zen Master's Guide to Redefining Power, Achieving True Freedom and Discovering Lasting Happiness in a Stressful World, by Thich Nhat Hanh

Peace Is Every Step, by Thich Nhat Hanh

The Headspace Guide to Meditation and Mindfulness, by Andy Puddicombe

Practicing Mindfulness: 75 Essential Meditations to Reduce Stress, Improve Mental Health, and Find Peace in the Everyday, by Matthew Sockolov

The Mindful Way Workbook: An 8-Week Program to Free Yourself from Depression and Emotional Distress, by John Teasdale, Mark Williams, and Zindel Segal

The Nature Fix: Why Nature Makes Us Happier, Healthier, and More Creative, by Florence Williams

Deeper Mindfulness, by Mark Williams and Danny Penman

Mindfulness: An Eight-Week Plan for Finding Peace in a Frantic World, by Mark Williams and Danny Penman

HOW TO FIND A SEX THERAPIST OR SEXUALITY COUNSELOR

American Association of Sexuality Educators, Counselors and Therapists (AASECT)
https://www.aasect.org

International Society for the Study of Women's Sexual Health (ISSWSH)
https://www.isswsh.org

Society for Sex Therapy and Research (SSTAR)
https://sstarnet.org

The Society for the Scientific Study of Sexuality (SSSS)
https://sexscience.org

WEBSITES

Here are some good websites that provide support and information to help patients and their loved ones manage the sexual side effects of cancer and its treatments.

American Cancer Society
Use the search term "sexuality" to find a variety of topics.
https://www.cancer.org

Dana-Farber Cancer Institute
https://www.dana-farber.org

Macmillan Cancer Support
https://www.macmillan.org.uk/cancer-information
-and-support/treatment/coping-with-treatment/your
-sex-life/sex-and-side-effects-of-cancer-treatment

MD Anderson Cancer Center
https://www.mdanderson.org

Memorial Sloan Kettering Cancer Center (MSKCC)
https://www.mskcc.org

OncoLink
https://www.oncolink.org/support/sexuality-fertility
/sexuality/men-sexual-health-and-cancer
https://www.oncolink.org/support/sexuality-fertility
/sexuality/women-sexual-health-and-cancer

Scientific Network on Female Sexual Health and Cancer
https://www.cancersexnetwork.org

PODCASTS

There are multiple podcasts about mindfulness meditation as well as coping with or surviving cancer. You'll find them on Apple Podcasts, Spotify, and other podcast apps.

Mindfulness:

10% Happier with Dan Harris
Hosted by ABC News anchor Dan Harris, this podcast explores mindfulness from a skeptical and relatable perspective. Harris interviews experts on how mindfulness can improve mental well-being.
https://www.meditatehappier.com/

The Mindful Minute
This podcast by Meryl Arnett offers short, focused guided meditations designed to fit into your daily routine. It's perfect for beginners or those with busy schedules.
https://www.merylarnett.com

Tara Brach
Tara Brach blends mindfulness meditation with Buddhist teachings and modern psychology. Her podcast includes both guided meditations and spiritual discussions.
https://www.tarabrach.com

Mindfulness Mode
Hosted by Bruce Langford, this interview-based podcast focuses on practical tips and personal stories related to mindfulness and meditation.
https://www.mindfulnessmode.com

The Daily Meditation Podcast
Mary Meckley guides listeners through short daily meditations aimed at cultivating mindfulness and managing anxiety, sleep issues, and stress.
https://podcasts.apple.com/us/podcast/daily-meditation-podcast/id892107837

The Breathwork Club
Each episode provides different breathing techniques to help with stress relief, better sleep, and increased energy levels.
https://podcasts.apple.com/us/podcast/the-breathwork-club/id1536333599

Cancer:

You, Me and the Big C
Hosted by cancer survivors, this podcast is known for its candid discussions about living with cancer, covering everything from treatment to dating after a diagnosis.
https://www.bbc.co.uk/programmes/p0608649/episodes/downloads

Cancer Horizons
This podcast focuses on the latest advancements in cancer therapies. It shares personal stories of survival, making complex medical topics more accessible.
https://www.curetoday.com/podcasts

*Cancer Actually F**king Sucks*
A gritty, honest take on surviving cancer, hosted by survivors who share the unfiltered realities of the cancer experience.

https://open.spotify.com/show/5akVsQrTKNHm
8bjp3tjihu

Cancer for Breakfast
This podcast feels like having a supportive chat with
friends who understand the cancer journey, blending
personal experiences with expert insights.
https://open.spotify.com/show/2WBhJrBZVYUt04UM
8mXbl3

Your Stories: Conquering Cancer
Focused on storytelling, this podcast features cancer
survivors sharing their journeys from diagnosis to
survival, providing inspiration to others.
https://www.conquer.org/impact/your-stories

Talking Cancer
Offering a platform for open discussions, this podcast
includes insights from survivors and health-care
experts about navigating life with cancer.
https://www.macmillan.org.uk/cancer-information
-and-support/diagnosis/talking-about-cancer/talking
-cancer-podcast

Black Women Rising—The Untold Cancer Stories
This podcast amplifies the voices of Black women
sharing their cancer experiences, creating a supportive
community for underrepresented survivors.
https://open.spotify.com/show/0A9blkabh296UQk
g9p35a5

Cancer Advances
Focused on the forefront of cancer research, this
podcast shares insights from medical experts and
updates on the latest treatments.
https://my.clevelandclinic.org/podcasts/cancer-advances

Cancer Buzz
Covering various aspects of cancer care, this podcast includes patient stories, health-care innovations, and policy discussions relevant to survivors. https://www.accc-cancer.org/podcast

APPS

Look for the following meditation and mental health apps for Apple and Android devices. Many of them have limited content available for free with additional content available for purchase.

Balance
https://balanceapp.com/

Calm
https://www.calm.com

Headspace
https://www.headspace.com

Healthy Minds
https://hminnovations.org/meditation-app

Insight Timer
https://insighttimer.com

Jon Kabat-Zinn
https://jkzmeditations.com/the-app/

Mindfulness Coach
https://mobile.va.gov/app/mindfulness-coach

Oxford Mindfulness
https://oxfordmindfulness.org/oxford-mindfulness -app

Smiling Mind
   https://www.smilingmind.com.au/smiling-mind-app

Website with recommendations for free meditation apps
   https://www.mindful.org/free-mindfulness-apps
   -worthy-of-your-attention/

Appendix 1
Mindfulness Meditation

Mindfulness meditation made its way into Western medicine through the practice and research of Jon Kabat-Zinn, a molecular biologist and author of multiple books (https://jonkabat-zinn.com). In the 1980s he also started the Center for Mindfulness at the University of Massachusetts. Over the years, practitioners have developed specific mindfulness meditation interventions to treat depression, anxiety, panic attacks, and nausea during chemotherapy treatments.

Here are two mindfulness-based exercises you may want to try.

1. Focus on the breath
   - With eyes closed and sitting comfortably on a chair or the floor, notice where your body meets the seat or the floor.
   - As you breathe, feel how air moves into your nose through your nostrils. Pay attention to the rest of your body as you breathe out.
   - Does your chest or stomach move as you breathe in and out?
   - Is your attention to the breath wavering?
   - Are you thinking about other things?
   - Move your attention back to your breath and continue to focus on your breathing.
   - Your mind will probably drift as you do this exercise. That's okay; *you are not failing this exercise.*

This exercise captures the essence of mindfulness—not judging how you are meditating and being in the moment.

2. The raisin exercise

Ideally, someone should slowly read these instructions to you as you work through the meditation. To do this exercise alone, search online for "Raisin Meditation," and you'll find videos and audio guides. You need a single raisin for this exercise.

- Hold the raisin on your palm or between your fingers.

- Look at the raisin closely. Notice its size and color, and the bumps and crevices on its surface.

- Notice whether it's shiny or dull, and how the light shines on it and changes its color.

- Smell the raisin; what does it smell like?

- Lift the raisin to your ear and rub it carefully between your fingers. Does it make a sound?

- Place the raisin against your lips with your mouth closed. How does it feel? How is your body reacting to the raisin that's so close to your mouth?

- Open your mouth and put the raisin on your tongue. Roll it around your mouth with your tongue. Don't bite it; notice how the raisin feels against your teeth, gums, and cheeks.

- Slowly take one single bite of the raisin; how does it taste?

- Slowly chew the raisin, noticing its texture and taste.

- Swallow the raisin and notice the sensation as it moves down your throat. Now focus on the taste that's left in your mouth.

- When a thought interrupts your focus on the raisin, don't give up. Pay attention to the thought or sensation and then bring your focus back to the raisin.

This exercise is usually done in a group setting with discussion afterward about how it felt to focus on the simple act of eating a single raisin this way.

If you'd like to read more about mindfulness, see chapter 13 for a list of books I recommend. In chapter 13, I also offer a list of meditation and mental health apps.

Appendix 2
Sensate Focus Exercises

Instructions for Couples

The purpose of doing sensate focus exercises is to connect you with your own body and its sensations.

- This is a mindful practice; pay attention to the sensations *you* experience without judgment or expectation.
- Focus on touch, temperature, pressure, and texture.
- This is meant to be *touch for yourself* rather than for your partner.
- If your mind wanders, bring your focus back to what you're feeling through touching your partner.
- Ignore thoughts about what your partner is feeling; this is about *you*.
- Schedule three sessions every week.
- Do not do the exercises at bedtime.

STAGE 1

In this stage, touching the breast(s), chest, and genitals is not allowed.

One person initiates the exercises and goes first.

Ensure that you won't be disturbed (no phones, no pets, door closed and locked).

Do not play music, light candles, or do anything else to suggest this exercise is romantic; this is about being mindful and connecting with your body in a sensual rather than sexual manner.

Keep the temperature in the room comfortable.

You may wear some clothes, but being naked is preferable; cover up as little as possible to be comfortable.

Assume any position that's comfortable for both you and your partner.

Each person touches long enough to practice focusing on sensations and managing distractions by refocusing on sensations, but not so long that you get bored or tired. Ten to fifteen minutes is enough time to get the benefits of the exercise, but try not to watch the clock.

Touch with hands (fingertips, palms, and back of hands), but do not kiss or make full body contact.

If the person being touched finds that one area is ticklish or uncomfortable, they can move the other person's hand away using gentle touch over the person's hand.

No talking is allowed other than when the person who is doing the touching wants to switch roles and be the one who is touched. Use the word "switch" to indicate it's time to switch roles.

STAGE 2

Once you both can touch with focus on the self and sensations, and without distraction, you can move on to the second stage, which allows touching the breast(s), chest, and genitals.

Begin with some time on non-erotic areas, as in stage 1, and then progress to stage 2.

Incorporate touching the breast(s), chest, or genitals with the same focus as in stage 1.

Don't focus solely on these areas; move back and forth between the rest of the body and the breast(s), chest, and genitals.

The person being touched can gently move the other person's hand if they feel uncomfortable with the area being touched.

If either partner becomes aroused, they should focus on those sensations and resist the temptation to "do" something about them (fall into previous behavior).

STAGE 3

In this stage, penetration of the vagina with a penis is allowed. Once again, at each session, start touching using stages 1 and 2, then progress to this final stage.

Use a silicone lubricant for penetration (this can be put on the penis or at the entrance to the vagina).

The woman on top or astride her partner is the preferred position so that she can control the depth of penetration.

Take it slow; you can stop at any time if you feel anxious, experience unpleasurable sensations, or experience pain.

Move your partner's hand away from the area where touch is not pleasurable. Do not swat your partner's hand away, and resist the temptation to move away or shout.

Modified and used with permission from Linda Weiner and Constance Avery-Clark, authors of *Sensate Focus in Sex Therapy: The Illustrated Manual*, Routledge, 2017.

Instructions for Women Who Experience Pain with Genital Touch or Penetration

STAGE 1

The first stage is for the woman to feel comfortable with touching herself and to focus on how it feels. This needs to be a conscious process—feel all the sensations!

This exercise needs to be done *daily*—in the bath or lying on your bed in private.

If you feel tense about doing the exercise, practice relaxation with meditation or deep breathing.

When you're ready, follow these three steps:

- Place your smallest finger at the entrance to the vagina *without* inserting it.
- Contract or tighten the muscles of the pelvic floor for a slow count of 1 . . . 2 . . . 3.
- Let go of the contraction or tightening.

Repeat these steps *three* times, then take a 10-second break.

Repeat this complete sequence *three* times (for a total of *nine* contractions) at least once a day (twice is better!).

Practice this *without* insertion until you notice that you're no longer uncomfortable.

You are now ready to begin inserting your smallest finger.

Repeat the sequence above for a total of *nine* contractions (with 10-second breaks) while slowly inserting your smallest finger just a tiny bit.

If you're able to tolerate this, then repeat the sequence above while inserting your finger a tiny bit more.

When you're comfortable inserting your smallest finger all the way into the vagina, it's time to use a larger finger, while repeating the sequence of contractions, relaxation, and breaks.

You can insert two, three, or four fingers as you progress.

STAGE 2

In the second stage, once you're comfortable with inserting something that's approximately the same circumference as your partner's penis, or a dildo if you're using one, you can move to the *sensate focus exercises for couples* if desired.

Modified and used with permission from Linda Weiner and Constance Avery-Clark, authors of *Sensate Focus in Sex Therapy: The Illustrated Manual*, Routledge, 2017.

References

Chapter 1. The Human Sexual Response

1. Masters, W. H., and V. Johnson. *Human Sexual Response*. Boston: Little, Brown; 1966.
2. Kaplan, H. S. *Disorders of Sexual Desire*. New York: Simon & Schuster; 1979.
3. Zilbergeld, B., and C. Ellison. Desire discrepancies and arousal problems in sex therapy. In: S. Leiblum and L. Pervin, eds. *Principles and Practice of Sex Therapy*. New York: Guilford Press; 1980. p. 65–101.
4. Basson, R. The female sexual response: a different model. *Journal of Sex & Marital Therapy*. 2000;26(0092–623; 1):51–65.
5. Nagoski, E. *Come as You Are*. New York: Simon & Schuster; 2015.
6. Katz, A., and D. S. Dizon. Sexuality after cancer: a model for male survivors. *J Sex Med*. 2016;13(1):70–78.

Chapter 2. "Who will want me when I look like this?"

1. Przezdziecki, A., K. A. Sherman, A. Baillie, A. Taylor, E. Foley, and K. Stalgis-Bilinski. My changed body: breast cancer, body image, distress and self-compassion. *Psychooncology*. 2013;22(8):1872–1879.

Chapter 3. "I have no interest in sex—will it ever come back?"

1. Duthie, C. J., H. J. Calich, C. M. Rapsey, and E. Wibowo. Maintenance of sexual activity following androgen deprivation in males. *Crit Rev Oncol Hematol*. 2020;153:103064.
2. Luo, F., M. Link, C. Grabenhorst, and B. Lynn. Low sexual desire in breast cancer survivors and patients: a review. *Sex Med Rev*. 2022;10(3):367–375.
3. Robinson, P. J., R. J. Bell, M. K. Christakis, S. R. Ivezic, and S. R. Davis. Aromatase inhibitors are associated with low sexual desire causing distress and fecal incontinence in women: an observational study. *J Sex Med*. 2017;14(12):1566–1574.

Chapter 4. "Nothing's happening down there"

1. Neal, D. E., et al. Ten-year mortality, disease progression, and treatment-related side effects in men with localised prostate cancer from the ProtecT randomised controlled trial according to treatment received. *Eur Urol*. 2020;77(3):320–330.

2. Damast, S., et al. Literature review of vaginal stenosis and dilator use in radiation oncology. *Practical Radiation Oncology*. 2019;9(6):479–491.

3. Barocas, D. A., et al. Association between radiation therapy, surgery, or observation for localized prostate cancer and patient-reported outcomes after 3 years. *JAMA*. 2017;317(11):1126–1140.

4. Feng, D., C. Tang, S. Liu, Y. Yang, P. Han, and W. Wei. Current management strategy of treating patients with erectile dysfunction after radical prostatectomy: a systematic review and meta-analysis. *Int J Impot Res*. 2022;34(1):18–36.

5. Lima, T. F. N., J. Bitran, F. S. Frech, and R. Ramasamy. Prevalence of post-prostatectomy erectile dysfunction and a review of the recommended therapeutic modalities. *Int J Impot Res*. 2021;33(4):401–409.

6. Bearelly, P., et al. Long-term intracavernosal injection therapy: treatment efficacy and patient satisfaction. *Int J Impot Res*. 2020;32(3):345–351.

7. Wang, V. M., and L. A. Levine. Safety and efficacy of inflatable penile prostheses for the treatment of erectile dysfunction: evidence to date. *Med Devices (Auckl)*. 2022;15:27–36.

Chapter 5. "What's the point if I feel nothing?"

1. Milbury, K., and H. Badr. Sexual problems, communication patterns, and depressive symptoms in couples coping with metastatic breast cancer. *Psychooncology*. 2013;22(4):814–822.

2. Blouet, A., et al. Sexual quality of life evaluation after treatment among women with breast cancer under 35 years old. *Support Care Cancer*. 2019;27(3):879–885.

3. Nagoski, E. *Come as You Are*. New York: Simon & Schuster; 2015.

Chapter 6. "It hurts—why is this happening?"

1. Frey, A., C. Pedersen, H. Lindberg, R. Bisbjerg, J. Sønksen, and M. Fode. Prevalence and predicting factors for commonly neglected sexual side effects to external-beam radiation therapy for prostate cancer. *J Sex Med*. 2017;14(4):558–565.

2. Towe, M., L. M. Huynh, F. El-Khatib, J. Gonzalez, L. C. Jenkins, and F. A. Yafi. A review of male and female sexual function following colorectal surgery. *Sex Med Rev*. 2019;7(3):422–429.

3. Alananzeh, I., et al. Sexual activity and cancer: a systematic review of prevalence, predictors and information needs among female Arab cancer survivors. *Eur J Cancer Care (Engl)*. 2022;31(6):e13644.

4. Barsky Reese, J., K. A. Sorice, L. A. Zimmaro, S. J. Lepore, and M. C. Beach. Communication about sexual health in breast cancer: what can we learn from patients' self-report and clinic dialogue? *Patient Educ Couns.* 2020;103(9):1821–1829.

Chapter 7. *"My world is gray—I hate this feeling"*

1. Maass, S.W., C. Roorda, A. J. Berendsen, P. F. M. Verhaak, and G. H. de Bock. The prevalence of long-term symptoms of depression and anxiety after breast cancer treatment: a systematic review. *Maturitas.* 2015;82(1):100–108.
2. Watts, S., P. Prescott, J. Mason, N. McLeod, and G. Lewith. Depression and anxiety in ovarian cancer: a systematic review and meta-analysis of prevalence rates. *BMJ Open.* 2015;5(11):e007618.
3. Watts, S., et al. A quantitative analysis of the prevalence of clinical depression and anxiety in patients with prostate cancer undergoing active surveillance. *BMJ Open.* 2015;5(5):e006674.
4. Patient health questionnaire-2. Stanford Medicine. October 6, 2016. https://med.stanford.edu/content/dam/sm/ppc/documents/Mental_Health/PHQ-2_English.pdf.
5. Barsky Reese, J., et al. Patient-provider communication about sexual concerns in cancer: a systematic review. *J Cancer Surviv.* 2017;11(2):175–188.
6. Kent, E. E., et al. Health information needs and health-related quality of life in a diverse population of long-term cancer survivors. *Patient Educ Couns.* 2012;89(2):345–352.
7. Andersen, B. L., et al. Management of anxiety and depression in adult survivors of cancer: ASCO guideline update. *Journal of Clinical Oncology.* 2023;0(0):JCO.23.00293.
8. Wang, X., et al. Prognostic value of depression and anxiety on breast cancer recurrence and mortality: a systematic review and meta-analysis of 282,203 patients. *Mol Psychiatry.* 2020;25(12):3186–3197.

Chapter 8. *"I can't take it anymore!"*

1. What is lung cancer? American Cancer Society. January 29, 2024. https://www.cancer.org/cancer/types/lung-cancer/about/what-is.html.
2. Treating non-small cell lung cancer. American Cancer Society. October 29, 2024. https://www.cancer.org/cancer/types/lung-cancer/treating-non-small-cell.html.

3. Sedrak, M. S., and H. J. Cohen. The aging-cancer cycle: mechanisms and opportunities for intervention. *J Gerontol A Biol Sci Med Sci.* 2023;78(7):1234–1238.

4. Abazari, A., S. Chatterjee, and M. Moniruzzaman. Understanding cancer caregiving and predicting burden: an analytics and machine learning approach. *AMIA Annu Symp Proc.* 2023;2023:243–252.

5. Key statistics for brain and spinal cord tumors. American Cancer Society. January 16, 2025. https://www.cancer.org/cancer/types/brain -spinal-cord-tumors-adults/about/key-statistics.html.

6. Lien, A. W., and G. Rohde. Coping in the role as next of kin of a person with a brain tumour: a qualitative metasynthesis. *BMJ Open.* 2022;12(9): e052872.

7. Zwinkels, H., et al. Prevalence of changes in personality and behavior in adult glioma patients: a systematic review. *Neurooncol Pract.* 2016;3(4):222–231.

8. Knowlton, S. E., A. I. Gundersen, J. M. Reilly, C. O. Tan, J. C. Schneider, and S. L. Shih. Predictors of acute transfer and mortality within 6 months from admission to an inpatient rehabilitation facility for patients with brain tumors. *Arch Phys Med Rehabil.* 2022;103(3):424–429.

9. Coolbrandt, A., et al. Family caregivers of patients with a high-grade glioma: a qualitative study of their lived experience and needs related to professional care. *Cancer Nurs.* 2015;38(5):406–413.

10. Forst, D. A., et al. Characterizing distress and identifying modifiable intervention targets for family caregivers of patients with malignant gliomas. *J Palliat Med.* 2023;26(1):17–27.

Chapter 9. *"I've been affected too!"*

1. Elias, L. J., and I. Abdus-Saboor. Bridging skin, brain, and behavior to understand pleasurable social touch. *Curr Opin Neurobiol.* 2022;73:102527.

2. Smith, D. R. The human touch. *EMBO Rep.* 2021;22(10):e53789.

3. Harris, E. Meta-analysis: touch tied to improved mental, physical health. *JAMA.* 2024;331(20):1699.

4. Burstein, H. J., et al. Adjuvant endocrine therapy for women with hormone receptor-positive breast cancer: American Society of Clinical Oncology clinical practice guideline update on ovarian suppression. *J Clin Oncol.* 2016;34(14):1689–1701.

5. Schick, V., et al. Sexual behaviors, condom use, and sexual health of Americans over 50: implications for sexual health promotion for older adults. *Journal of Sexual Medicine.* 2010;7:315–329.

6. Berkowitz, M. J., et al. How patients experience endocrine therapy for breast cancer: an online survey of side effects, adherence, and medical team support. *Journal of Cancer Survivorship*. 2020.

7. Franzoi, M. A., et al. Evidence-based approaches for the management of side-effects of adjuvant endocrine therapy in patients with breast cancer. *Lancet Oncol.* 2021;22(7):e303–e313.

8. Akkuzu, G., and A. Ayhan. Sexual functions of Turkish women with gynecologic cancer during the chemotherapy process. *Asian Pac J Cancer Prev.* 2013;14(6):3561–3564.

9. Gray, T. F., D. R. Azizoddin, and P. V. Nersesian. Loneliness among cancer caregivers: a narrative review. *Palliat Support Care.* 2020;18(3):359–367.

10. Neal, D. E., et al. Ten-year mortality, disease progression, and treatment-related side effects in men with localised prostate cancer from the ProtecT randomised controlled trial according to treatment received. *Eur Urol.* 2020;77(3):320–330.

11. Barocas, D. A., et al. Association between radiation therapy, surgery, or observation for localized prostate cancer and patient-reported outcomes after 3 years. *JAMA.* 2017;317(11):1126–1140.

12. Nascimento, B., E. P. Miranda, L. C. Jenkins, N. Benfante, E. A. Schofield, and J. P. Mulhall. Testosterone recovery profiles after cessation of androgen deprivation therapy for prostate cancer. *Journal of Sexual Medicine.* 2019;16(6):872–879.

Chapter 10. *"I miss touching her"*

1. Siegel, R. L., A. N. Giaquinto, and A. Jemal. Cancer statistics, 2024. *CA: A Cancer Journal for Clinicians.* 2024;74(1):12–49.

2. Mulville, A. K., N. N. Widick, and N. S. Makani. Timely referral to hospice care for oncology patients: a retrospective review. *Am J Hosp Palliat Care.* 2019;36(6):466–471.

3. Sharafi, S., A. Ziaee, and H. Dahmardeh. What are the outcomes of hospice care for cancer patients? A systematic review. *Support Care Cancer.* 2022;31(1):64.

4. Malta, S., and I. Wallach. Sexuality and ageing in palliative care environments? Breaking the (triple) taboo. *Australas J Ageing.* 2020;39 Suppl 1:71–73.

5. Donz, R., et al. What contributes to promote sexual health in cancer palliative care? A realist review. *Sex Med Rev.* 2024;12(3):334–345.

6. McClelland, S. I. "I wish I'd known": patients' suggestions for supporting sexual quality of life after diagnosis with metastatic breast cancer. *Sexual and Relationship Therapy.* 2016;31(4):414–431.

7. Lemieux, L., S. Kaiser, J. Pereira, and L. M. Meadows. Sexuality in palliative care: patient perspectives. *Palliative Medicine*. 2004;18(0269–2163; 7):630–637.

8. Ussher, J. M., W. K. Tim Wong, and J. Perz. A qualitative analysis of changes in relationship dynamics and roles between people with cancer and their primary informal carer. *Health (London)*. 2011;15(6):650–667.

9. Valenti, K. G., S. Jen, J. Parajuli, A. Arbogast, A. L. Jacobsen, and S. Kunkel. Experiences of palliative and end-of-life care among older LGBTQ women: a review of current literature. *J Palliat Med*. 2020;23(11):1532–1539.

10. Berkman, C., G. L. Stein, D. Godfrey, N. M. Javier, S. Maingi, and S. O'Mahony. Disrespectful and inadequate palliative care to lesbian, gay, and bisexual patients. *Palliat Support Care*. 2023;21(5):782–787.

11. Haviland, K. S., S. Swette, T. Kelechi, and M. Mueller. Barriers and facilitators to cancer screening among LGBTQ individuals with cancer. *Oncol Nurs Forum*. 2020;47(1):44–55.

Chapter 11. Communication

1. Herbenick, D., M. Reece, V. Schick, S. A. Sanders, B. Dodge, and J. D. Fortenberry. Sexual behavior in the United States: results from a national probability sample of men and women ages 14–94. *Journal of Sexual Medicine*. 2010;7:255–265.

2. Dai, Y., O. Y. Cook, L. Yeganeh, C. Huang, J. Ding, and C. E. Johnson. Patient-reported barriers and facilitators to seeking and accessing support in gynecologic and breast cancer survivors with sexual problems: a systematic review of qualitative and quantitative studies. *J Sex Med*. 2020;17(7):1326–1358.

3. Ezhova, I., L. Savidge, C. Bonnett, J. Cassidy, A. Okwuokei, and T. Dickinson. Barriers to older adults seeking sexual health advice and treatment: a scoping review. *International Journal of Nursing Studies*. 2020;107:103566.

4. Fan, R., L. Wang, X. Bu, W. Wang, and J. Zhu. Unmet supportive care needs of breast cancer survivors: a systematic scoping review. *BMC Cancer*. 2023;23(1):587.

5. Kent, E. E., C. W. Wheldon, A. W. Smith, S. Srinivasan, and A. M. Geiger. Care delivery, patient experiences, and health outcomes among sexual and gender minority patients with cancer and survivors: a scoping review. *Cancer*. 2019;125(24):4371–4379.

6. Perez, G. K., J. M. Salsman, K. Fladeboe, A. C. Kirchhoff, E. R. Park, and A. R. Rosenberg. Taboo topics in adolescent and young adult oncology: strategies for managing challenging but important conversations central to adolescent and young adult cancer survivorship. *Am Soc Clin Oncol Educ Book.* 2020;40:1–15.
7. Pimsen, A., W. Lin, C. Lin, Y. Kuo, and B. Shu. Healthcare providers' experiences in providing sexual health care to breast cancer survivors: a mixed-methods systematic review. *J Clin Nurs.* 2024;33(3):797–816.
8. Kotronoulas, G., C. Papadopoulou, and E. Patiraki. Nurses' knowledge, attitudes, and practices regarding provision of sexual health care in patients with cancer: critical review of the evidence. *Support Care Cancer.* 2009;17(5):479–501.
9. Leonardi-Warren, K., I. Neff, M. Mancuso, B. Wenger, M. Galbraith, and R. Fink. Sexual health: exploring patient needs and healthcare provider comfort and knowledge. *Clinical Journal of Oncology Nursing.* 2016;20(6):E162–E167.
10. O'Connor, S. R., et al. Healthcare professional perceived barriers and facilitators to discussing sexual wellbeing with patients after diagnosis of chronic illness: a mixed-methods evidence synthesis. *Patient Educ Couns.* 2019;102(5):850–863.
11. Katz, A. *Woman Cancer Sex.* 2nd ed. New York: Routledge; 2021. p. 180.

Chapter 12. Lotions, Pills, and Potions

1. Dos Santos, B. S., C. Bordignon, and D. D. Rosa. Managing common estrogen deprivation side effects in HR+ breast cancer: an evidence-based review. *Curr Oncol Rep.* 2021;23(6):63.
2. Cullen, K., K. Fergus, T. Dasgupta, M. Fitch, C. Doyle, and L. Adams. From "sex toy" to intrusive imposition: a qualitative examination of women's experiences with vaginal dilator use following treatment for gynecological cancer. *J Sex Med.* 2012;9(4):1162–1173.
3. Matos, S. R. L., M. L. R. Cunha, S. Podgaec, E. Weltman, A. F. Y. Centrone, and A. C. C. N. Mafra. Consensus for vaginal stenosis prevention in patients submitted to pelvic radiotherapy. *PLoS One.* 2019;14(8): e0221054.
4. Cyr, M. P., et al. Feasibility, acceptability and effects of multimodal pelvic floor physical therapy for gynecological cancer survivors suffering from painful sexual intercourse: a multicenter prospective interventional study. *Gynecol Oncol.* 2020;159(3):778–784.

5. Jha, S., L. Wyld, and P. H. Krishnaswamy. The impact of vaginal laser treatment for genitourinary syndrome of menopause in breast cancer survivors: a systematic review and meta-analysis. *Clin Breast Cancer.* 2019;19(4):e556–e562.

6. Brotto, L. A., et al. A psychoeducational intervention for sexual dysfunction in women with gynecologic cancer. *Archives of Sexual Behavior.* 2008;37:317–329.

7. Brotto, L. A., et al. A brief mindfulness-based cognitive behavioral intervention improves sexual functioning versus wait-list control in women treated for gynecologic cancer. *Gynecologic oncology.* 2012;125(2):320–325.

8. Mension, E., I. Alonso, and C. Castelo-Branco. Genitourinary syndrome of menopause: current treatment options in breast cancer survivors—systematic review. *Maturitas.* 2021;143:47–58.

9. Biglia, N., et al. Vaginal atrophy in breast cancer survivors: attitude and approaches among oncologists. *Clin Breast Cancer.* 2017;17(8):611–617.

10. Pavlović, R. T., et al. The safety of local hormonal treatment for vulvovaginal atrophy in women with estrogen receptor-positive breast cancer who are on adjuvant aromatase inhibitor therapy: meta-analysis. *Clin Breast Cancer.* 2019;19(6):e731–e740.

11. Pingarron, C., P. de Lafuente, A. M. Ierullo, S. P. Torcal, C. J. M. Díaz, and S. Palacios. Ospemifene in clinical practice for vulvo-vaginal atrophy: results at 3 months of follow-up of use. *Gynecol Endocrinol.* 2021;37(6): 562–566.

12. Cai, B., et al. No increase in incidence or risk of recurrence of breast cancer in ospemifene-treated patients with vulvovaginal atrophy (VVA). *Maturitas.* 2020;142:38–44.

13. Febrina, F., I. F. Triyoga, M. White, J. L. Marino, and M. Peate. Efficacy of interventions to manage sexual dysfunction in women with cancer: a systematic review. *Menopause.* 2022;29(5):609–626.

14. Barton, D. L., et al. Systemic and local effects of vaginal dehydroepiandrosterone (DHEA): NCCTG N10C1 (Alliance). *Support Care Cancer.* 2018;26(4):1335–1343.

15. Jaderek, I., and M. Lew-Starowicz. A systematic review on mindfulness meditation-based interventions for sexual dysfunctions. *J Sex Med.* 2019;16(10):1581–1596.

16. Gunst, A., et al. A randomized, waiting-list-controlled study shows that brief, mindfulness-based psychological interventions are effective for treatment of women's low sexual desire. *J Sex Res.* 2019;56(7):913–929.

17. Stephenson, K. R., N. Zippan, and L. A. Brotto. Feasibility of a cognitive behavioral online intervention for women with sexual interest/arousal disorder. *Journal of Clinical Psychology.* 2021;77(9):1877–1893.

18. Streicher, L., and J. A. Simon. Sexual function post-breast cancer. *Cancer Treat Res.* 2018; 73:167–189.

19. Bartlik, B., A. Sugarman, S. Seenaraine, and S. Green. FDA-approved (bremelanotide, flibanserin) and off-label medications (testosterone, sildenafil) to enhance sexual desire/function in women. *Online Journal of Complementary and Alternative Medicine.* 2020;4(1).

20. Pettigrew, J. A., and A. M. Novick. Hypoactive sexual desire disorder in women: physiology, assessment, diagnosis, and treatment. *J Midwifery Women's Health.* 2021;66(6):740–748.

21. Lorenz, T., J. Rullo, and S. Faubion. Antidepressant-induced female sexual dysfunction. *Mayo Clin Proc.* 2016;91(9):1280–1286.

22. Feng, D., C. Tang, S. Liu, Y. Yang, P. Han, and W. Wei. Current management strategy of treating patients with erectile dysfunction after radical prostatectomy: a systematic review and meta-analysis. *Int J Impot Res.* 2022;34(1):18–36.

23. Raina, R., G. Pahlajani, A. Agarwal, and C. D. Zippe. The early use of transurethral alprostadil after radical prostatectomy potentially facilitates an earlier return of erectile function and successful sexual activity. *BJU International.* 2007;100(6):1317–1321.

24. Bearelly, P., et al. Long-term intracavernosal injection therapy: treatment efficacy and patient satisfaction. *Int J Impot Res.* 2020;-32(3):345–351.

25. Lima, T. F. N., J. Bitran, F. S. Frech, and R. Ramasamy. Prevalence of post-prostatectomy erectile dysfunction and a review of the recommended therapeutic modalities. *Int J Impot Res.* 2021;33(4): 401–409.

26. Wang, V. M., and L. A. Levine. Safety and efficacy of inflatable penile prostheses for the treatment of erectile dysfunction: evidence to date. *Med Devices (Auckl).* 2022;15:27–36.

27. Jo, J. K., et al. Effect of starting penile rehabilitation with sildenafil immediately after robot-assisted laparoscopic radical prostatectomy on erectile function recovery: a prospective randomized trial. *J Urol.* 2018;199(6):1600–1606.

28. Sari Motlagh, R., et al. Penile rehabilitation strategy after nerve sparing radical prostatectomy: a systematic review and network meta-analysis of randomized trials. *J Urol.* 2021;205(4):1018–1030.

29. Albaugh, J., B. Adamic, C. Chang, N. Kirwen, and J. Aizen. Adherence and barriers to penile rehabilitation over 2 years following radical prostatectomy. *BMC Urol.* 2019;19(1):89.

30. Raheem, O. A., et al. Novel treatments of erectile dysfunction: review of the current literature. *Sexual Medicine Reviews.* 2020.

31. Baccaglini, W., et al. PS-5-9 erectile dysfunction after radical prostatectomy: low-intensity extracorporeal shockwave therapy (LIESWT) plays a role? *Journal of Sexual Medicine.* 2020;17(6):S136.

32. Wittmann, D., S. Foley, and R. Balon. A biopsychosocial approach to sexual recovery after prostate cancer surgery: the role of grief and mourning. *Journal of Sex and Marital Therapy.* 2011;37:130–144.

33. Geraerts, I., H. Van Poppel, N. Devoogdt, A. De Groef, S. Fieuws, and M. Van Kampen. Pelvic floor muscle training for erectile dysfunction and climacturia 1 year after nerve sparing radical prostatectomy: a randomized controlled trial. *Int J Impot Res.* 2016;28(1):9–13.

34. Kannady, C., and J. Clavell-Hernández. Orgasm-associated urinary incontinence (climacturia) following radical prostatectomy: a review of pathophysiology and current treatment options. *Asian J Androl.* 2020;22(6):549–554.

Index

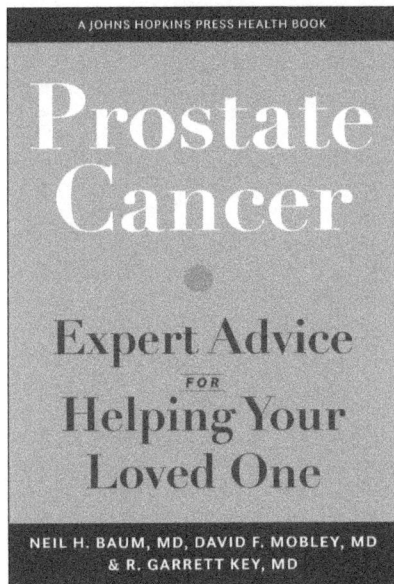

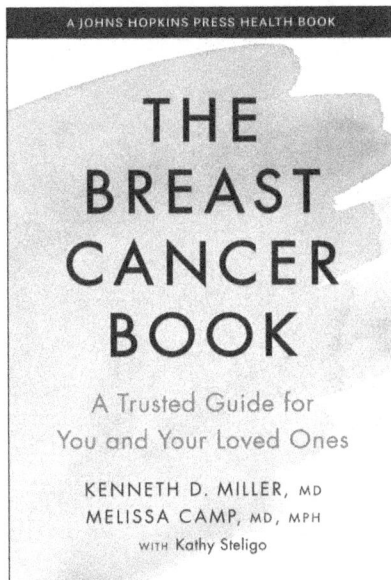

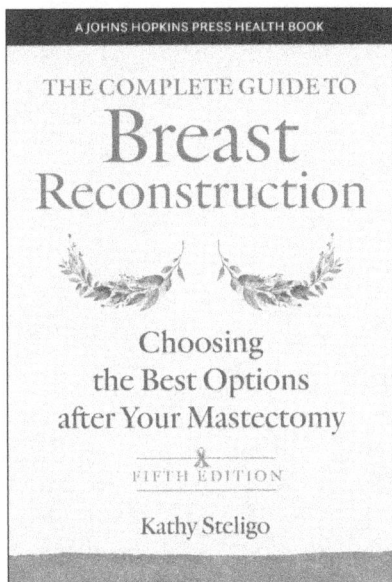

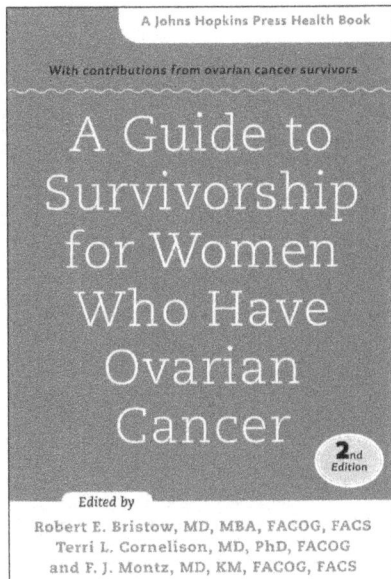